The Gluten-Free Sourdough Cookbook

gluten-free and dairy-free recipes
for everyday baking

by Kasey Lobb, MS, RDN

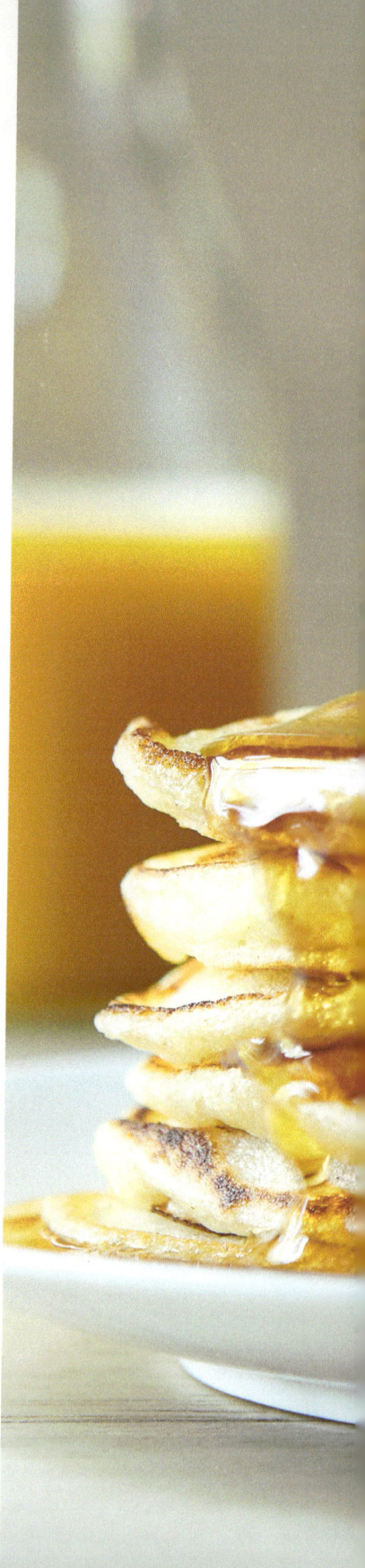

The Gluten-Free Sourdough Cookbook: gluten-free and dairy-free recipes for everyday baking
Written by Kasey Lobb, MS, RDN

Copyright© 2025

Published by Appetite to Travel, LLC

Year published: 2025
ISBN: 979-8-218-63058-4
Library of Congress Control Number: 2025906232

Cover and book design by Rae Zurcher
Photography by Jason Gamble
Food styling by Rae Zurcher and Kasey Lobb.

Printed in United States of America

Cover image: Simple Boule

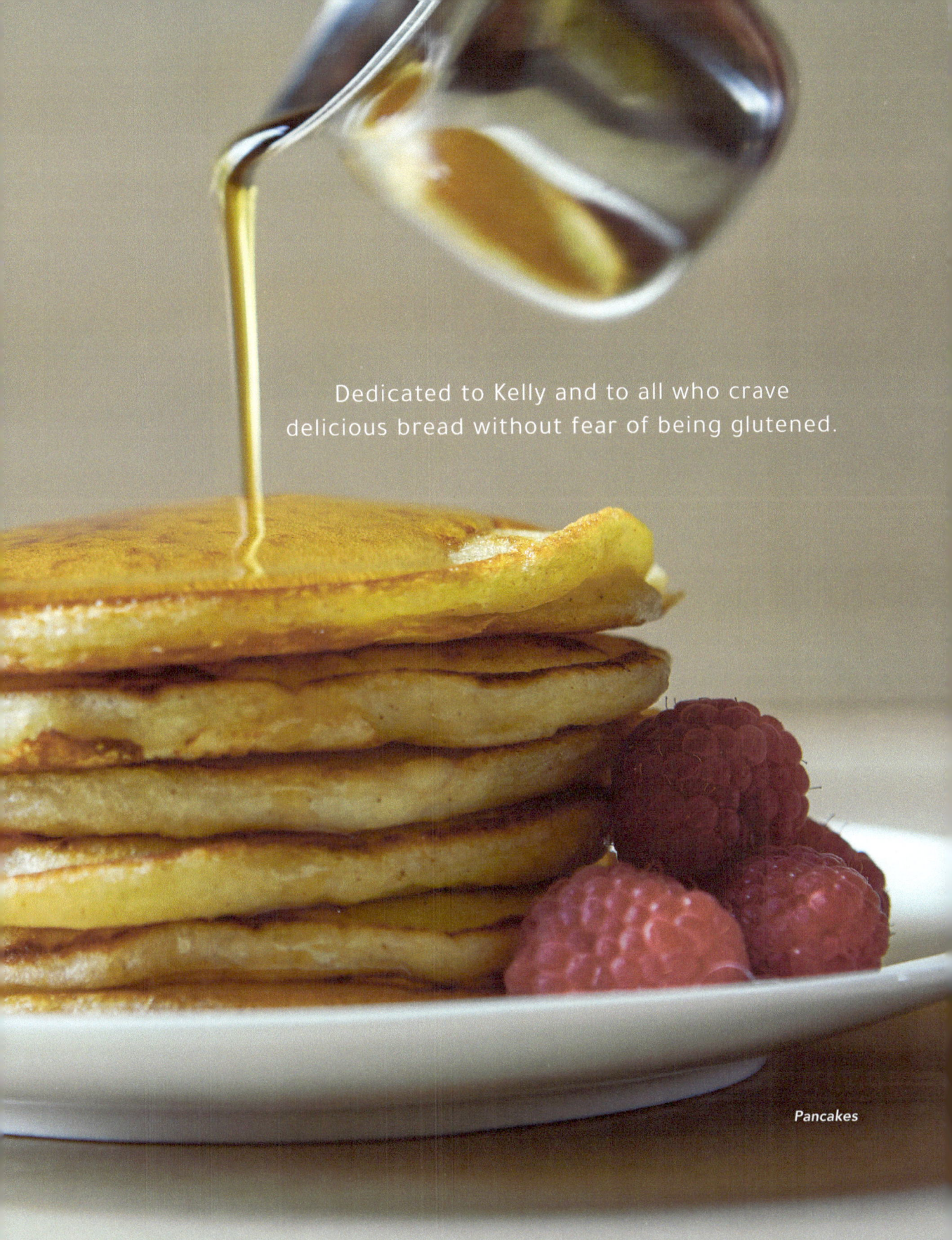

Dedicated to Kelly and to all who crave
delicious bread without fear of being glutened.

Pancakes

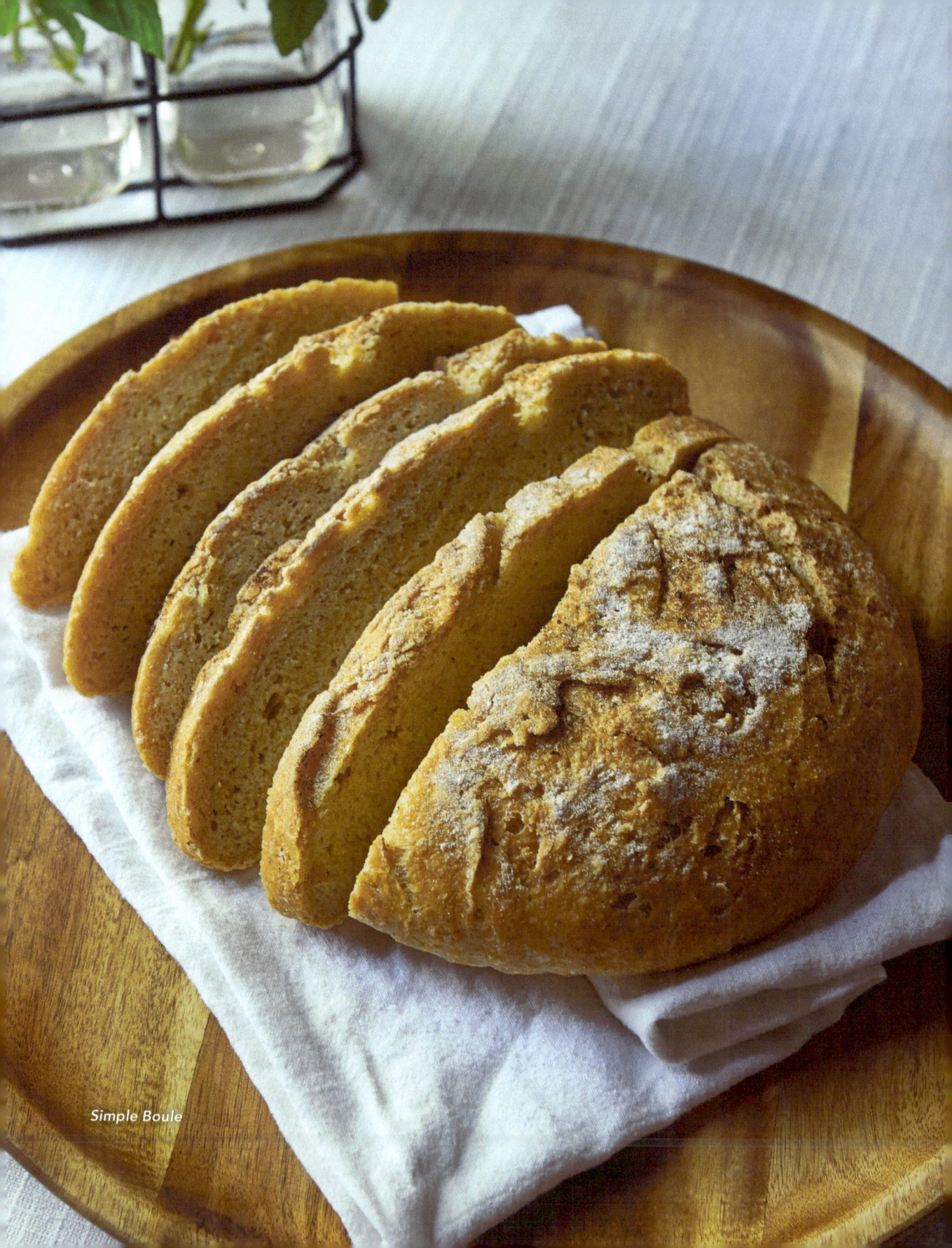

Simple Boule

Give us today our daily bread.

Matthew 6:11

Table of Contents

Introduction

I have a pocket-sized sourdough cookery book from 1977 that belonged to my mom. It still has the original B. Dalton price tag on the front, $2.95. Inside, you'll find doodles and drawings in my 5- or 6-year-old handwriting, along with mom's beautiful cursive notes – "try" and "make again!" Much has changed since the 70's, but the reasons my mom turned to that cookbook still hold true today. Baking heartwarming sourdough treats was her way of sharing the wonders of good nutrition. We still know that making foods at home is a practical and economical way to avoid preservatives and inflammatory additives. Plus, the naturally occurring yeast in sourdough helps break down grains and starches, making them easier to digest. These benefits of fermentation translate directly to crafting sourdough as gluten-free. As a dietitian and plant-based chef, I've refined the techniques needed to help you create gluten-free sourdough in your home.

Sometimes, the gluten-free lifestyle chooses you. Not everyone freely chooses to eat gluten-free, but everyone can benefit from taking a "gluten holiday." From autoimmune diseases to gut sensitivity, people follow a gluten-free diet for many health reasons and come to find store-bought gluten-free breads to be expensive, pasty and bland. The recipes in this gluten-free book are designed to look and taste as good as traditional wheat-based ones. However, the approach to achieving familiar results is much different. Gluten-free flours perform differently than wheat flour; they are lighter, heavier or stickier. The solution is to use a blend of at least three different gluten-free flours and starches. I've included a glossary of flours to help you navigate the nuances of gluten-free flour.

As a dietitian, I know store-bought gluten-free products rely on highly refined and processed flours that lack the nutritional value of whole grains. Eating these breads can lead to blood sugar imbalances. As a chef, I counter this by incorporating whole grains, nuts and seeds whenever possible without compromising the spirit of the final product. Milled nuts, seeds and legumes not only add nutrition but can improve texture and flavor. However, this is not a health book. My aim is to provide gluten- and dairy-free recipes that you will use often, and to share important tips and techniques so you can succeed in your kitchen.

This cookbook isn't filled with recipes you'll never try. Each one is designed to be useful in your menu planning and weekly meals. With straightforward instructions, these recipes are suited for all experience levels. All bakers benefit from the

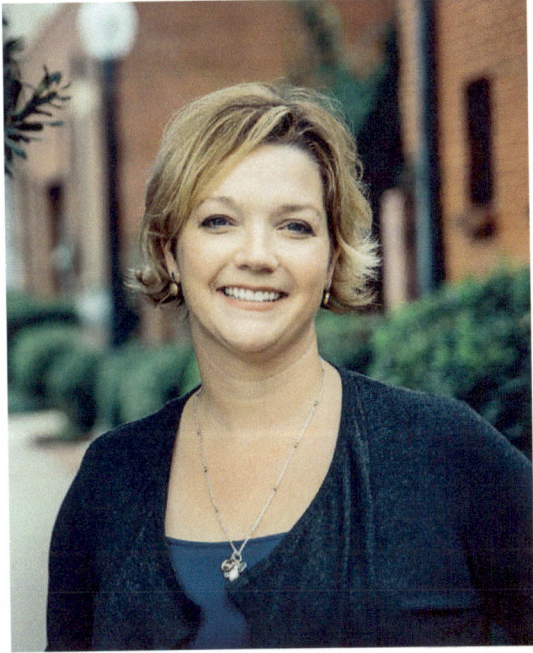

added descriptions and notes detailing how the recipe should look as you go along. To increase accessibility, I avoid using hard-to-find ingredients and I repeat ingredients across recipes. This helps keep a well-stocked pantry and refrigerator that is ready when you get the urge to bake.

Additionally, students in my cooking classes often mention that using a kitchen scale feels intimidating and is a barrier to baking at home. That's why this book focuses on using Imperial measuring utensils, just like my mom and Granny used. Be sure to review the **Get Started** chapter before you start, as it explains how to achieve scale-accurate results with measuring cups. So, you can get started with ingredients and tools already in your kitchen. I believe these recipes will become staples in your home. As you gain experience, I encourage you to make them your own!

See you in the kitchen,

Kasey

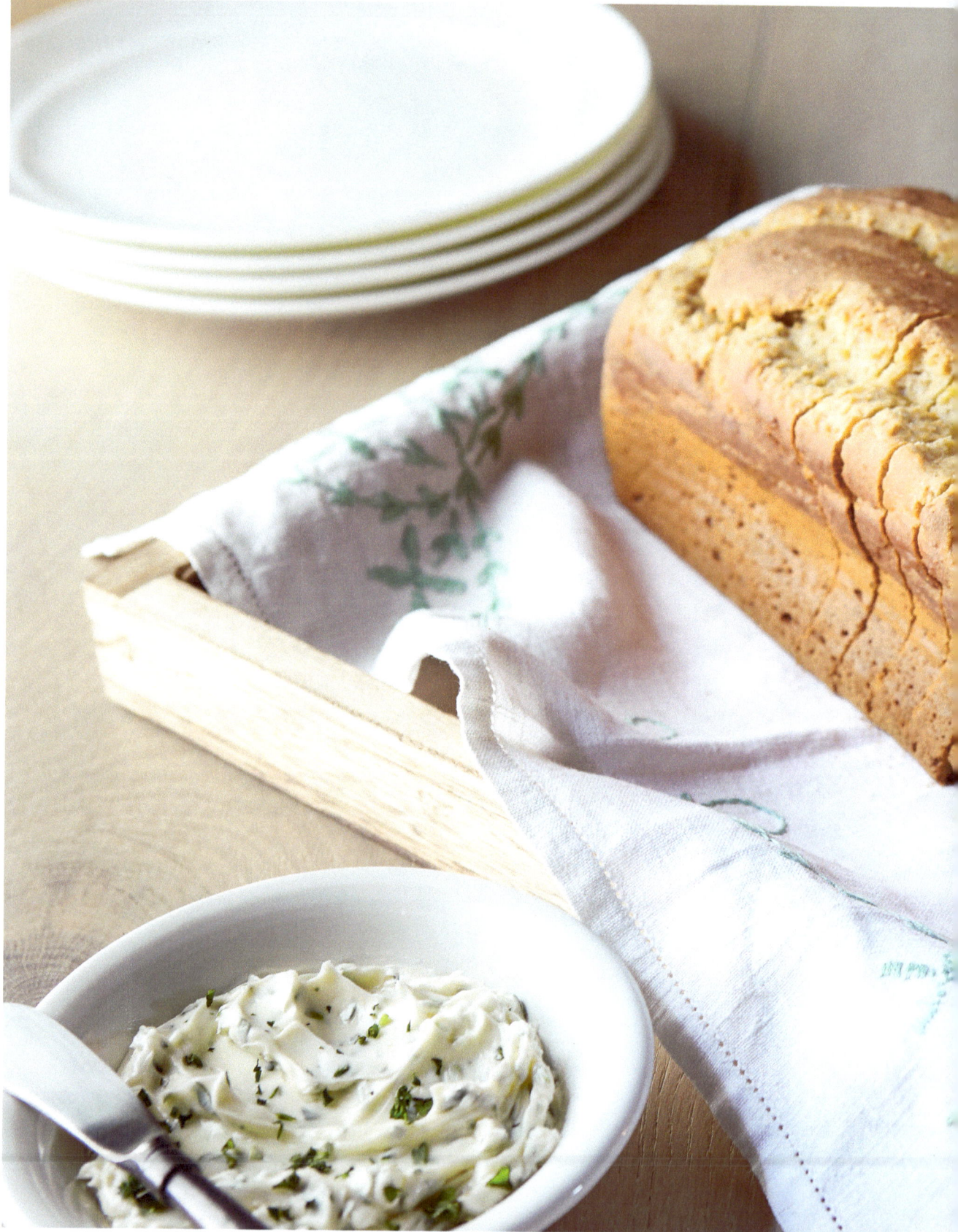

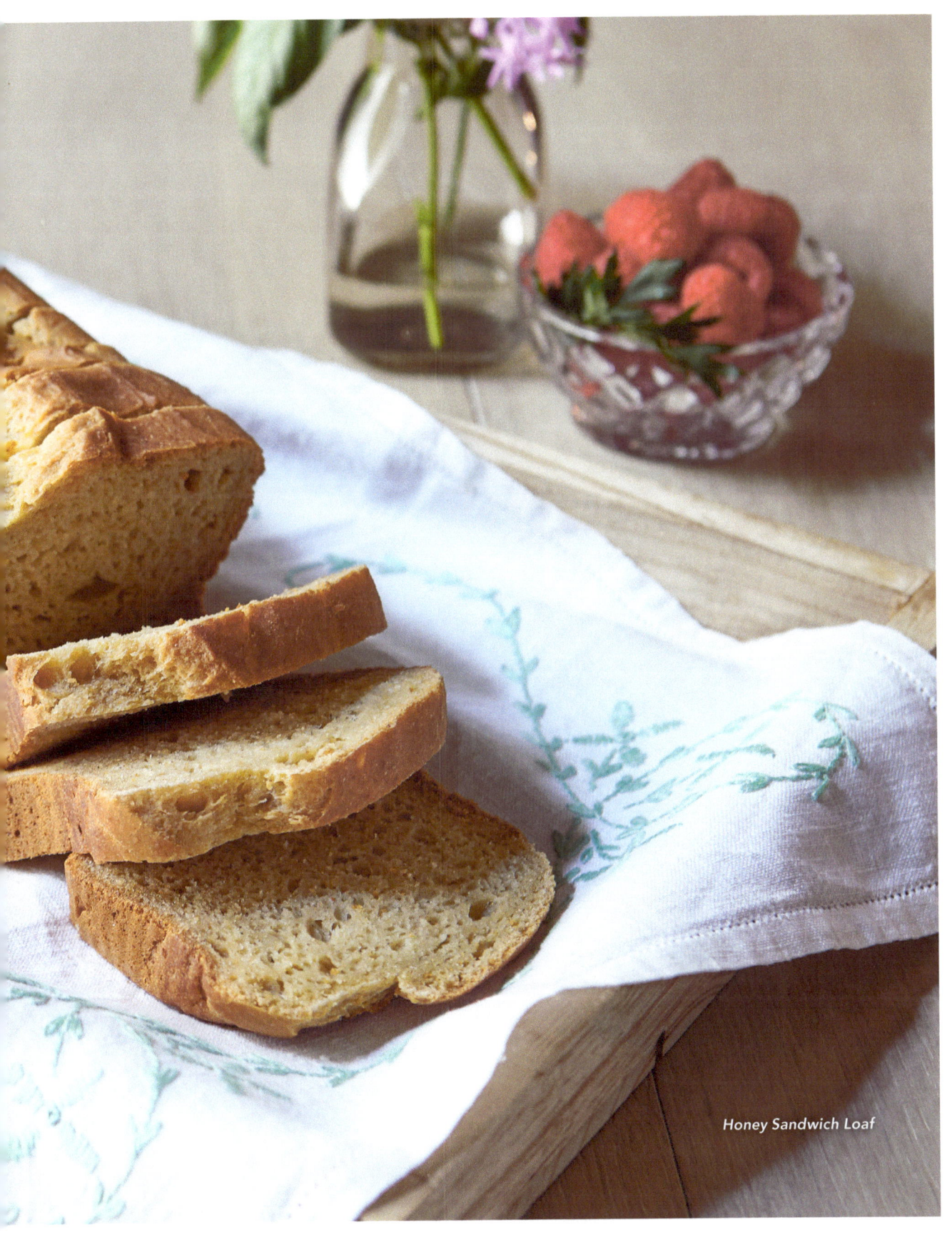

Honey Sandwich Loaf

Notes to the Baker

Gluten-free breads and treats act differently than their glutenous cousins, so don't be surprised if ingredients and instructions look or feel a little different. Roll with it!

No kitchen scale required – simply use your standard measuring cups, just like mom did.

Use any milk alternative, I recommend an **unsweetened** variety for best results. Where salt is listed, I suggest fine crystal sea salt.

I prefer a high-sided Pullman loaf pan. Cool loaf just enough to handle, run a knife around the sides, then cool completely on a wire rack before slicing.

Slicing gluten-free bread while still warm makes it lose loft and dry out.

If you already have a gluten-free starter, please review **Foundations of Baking Gluten-Free Sourdough** (p. 16) before baking.

If you are new to gluten-free sourdough, don't worry! **Get Started** has a day-by-day guide on how to grow starter and in-depth details on care and maintenance.

Most recipes in this book are forgiving when it comes to substitutions – even mistakes. If you are new to baking, start with a Pancake or the Coffee Cake recipe. Then try one of the **Quick Breads**.

The **Get Started** chapter and the **Glossaries** have answers to almost any question that might pop up. I'm cheering you on!

All recipes use unfed gluten-free starter. Just stir and measure.

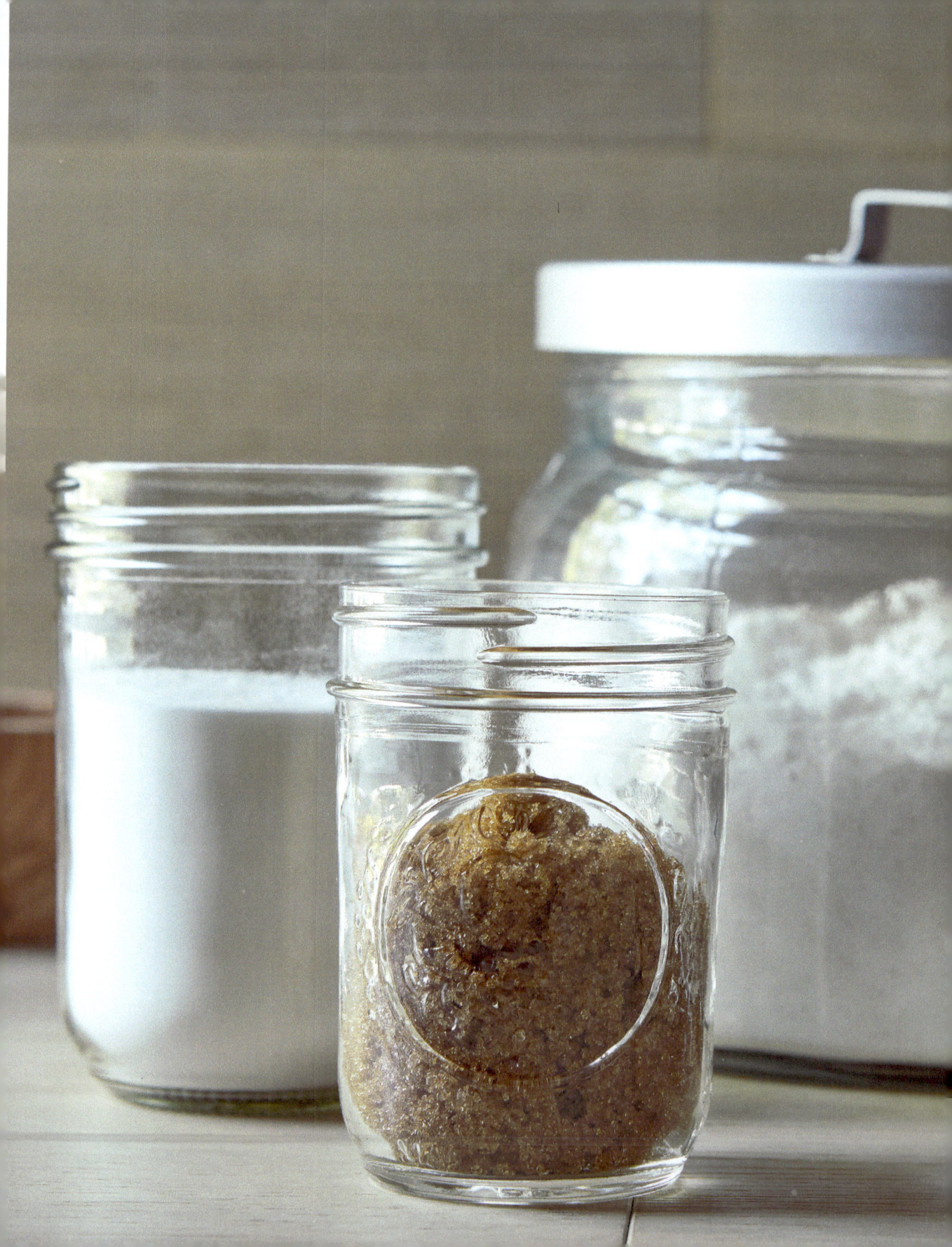

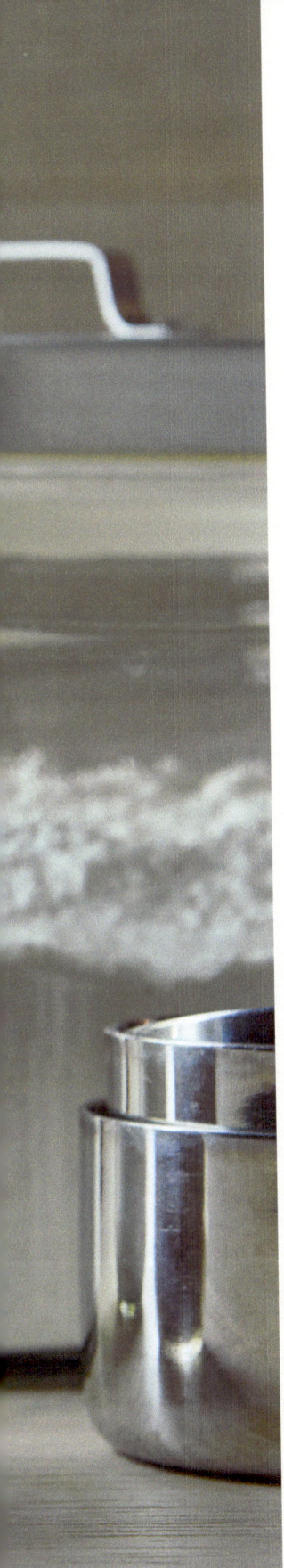

Get Started

There is a sweet sort of attachment that grows between you and your sourdough starter. Like me, you may soon be calling your gluten-free sourdough starter "mother". The oldest mother I've met was in Ireland a decade ago. The baking instructor said she was at least seven years old, but their previous mother had been started by his actual mother some twenty years earlier. My mother is now over six years old. She is a source of personal pride. I spent a year of experiments and failures before finally growing and maintaining her as a robust gluten-free sourdough starter.

Take time to study this chapter and even make use of the lined **Notes** pages in the back. I've packed this chapter with the foundational knowledge you need to master gluten-free sourdough baking. Whether you're new to gluten-free baking or looking to elevate your skills, you'll find tips, techniques, and key insights to set you up for success.

Most importantly, you'll learn how to grow and nurture your very own gluten-free mother. The mother is the true and flavorful heart of creating each recipe in this book. Your journey to gluten-free sourdough baking with confidence and success starts here, with growing your very own mother!

What is Sourdough?

Sourdough starter is a living culture created by harnessing natural yeast present in the air. The process of regular feeding and discarding over several days builds a thriving colony of wild yeast and beneficial bacteria. This healthy mixture provides leavening power for our sourdough bread and other baked goods, giving them a soft texture and distinctive tangy flavor. Unlike commercial yeast which is typically a single strain of yeast and works quickly and consistently, sourdough relies on a diverse community of yeasts and beneficial bacteria. This leads to a slower fermentation process that develops rich flavors and complex textures.

Making gluten-free sourdough goods present unique challenges due to the absence of gluten, which traditionally gives dough strong structure. To overcome this, gluten-free sourdough recipes use a blend of gluten-free flours, each contributing unique texture and flavor. The beauty of gluten-free sourdough lies in its natural and time-honored process, connecting bakers to a centuries-old tradition of baking, while also offering allergy-friendly treats for modern health needs.

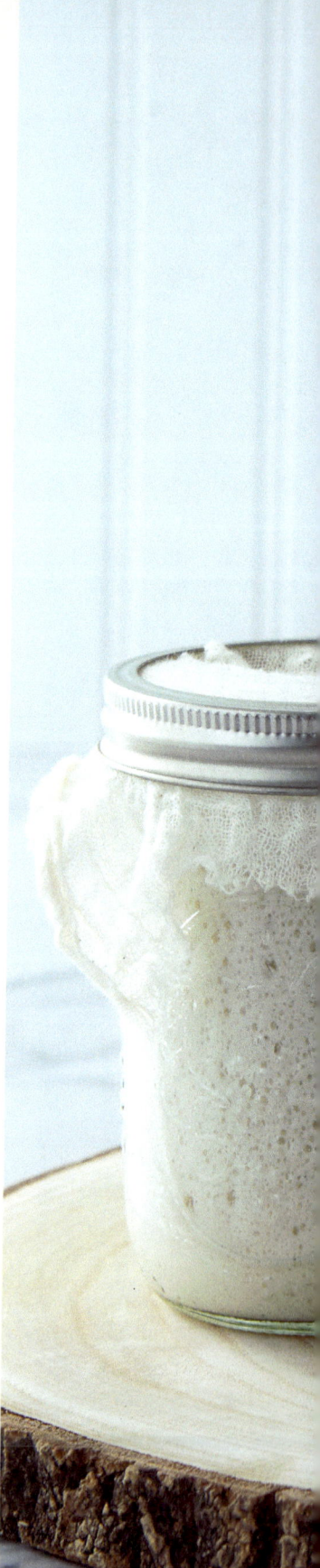

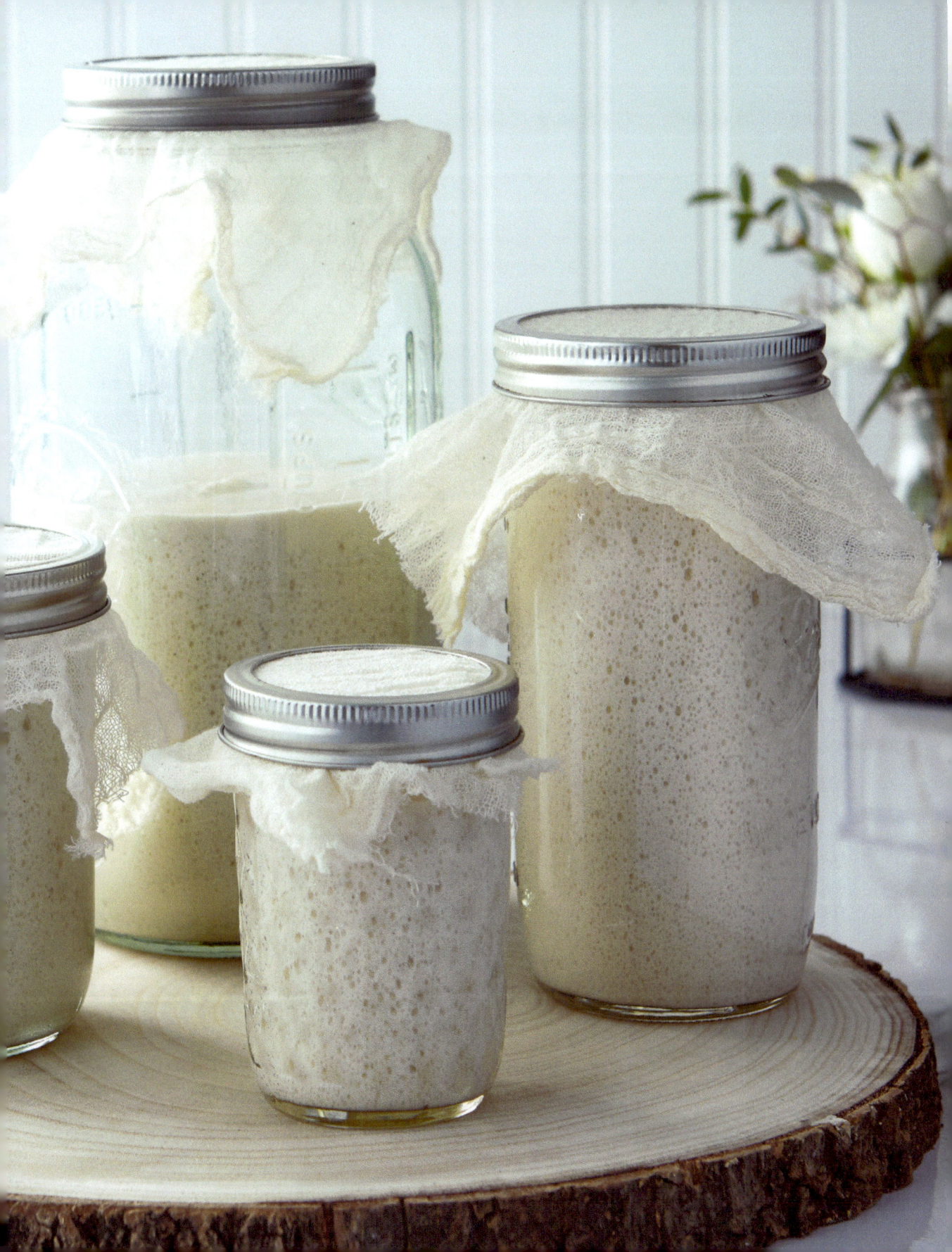

Foundations of Baking Gluten-Free Sourdough

Read the recipe completely before starting. Measure and lay out all ingredients – the French call this mise en place. This technique saves time and reduces recipe errors.

Measure flours and liquids according to **Measuring Techniques** (p. 20). Measuring cups for liquids are different than for dry ingredients (see p. 101).

Maintain a healthy kitchen: clean hands, clean jars and utensils before tending to your sourdough starter, avoid harsh and toxic chemicals, install proper thermometers in your oven, refrigerator and freezer (see **Kitchen and Pantry Guide**, p. 99).

Homemade gluten-free goods have a short shelf life. For best results, plan to freeze leftovers on the same day baked. Single-serving portions make it easy to thaw and reheat. Storing in airtight container maintains high quality.

Gluten-Free Baking Tips

A **highly active starter** is one that creates bubbling, even under refrigeration, within 4 hours of feeding.

Wash hands and all utensils well before each use to minimize chance of unwanted contamination.

Always **stir sourdough starter before measuring** for a recipe using clean utensils.

These recipes accommodate a wide range of starter consistencies, but in general, starters should resemble **thick pancake batter**. A thin starter is more hydrated than a thicker starter and over time you can learn to adjust the recipe to accommodate conditions of the starter.

Recipes with gluten-free flours benefit greatly from **20 to 30-minutes rest before baking** to fully hydrate the starches.

Sourdough starter adds moisture to a recipe. Take notice of the starter's hydration and activity. The amount of sourdough starter used in a recipe can increase baking time.

Remove gluten-free bread from pan to a wire rack to prevent condensation that can make bread soggy.

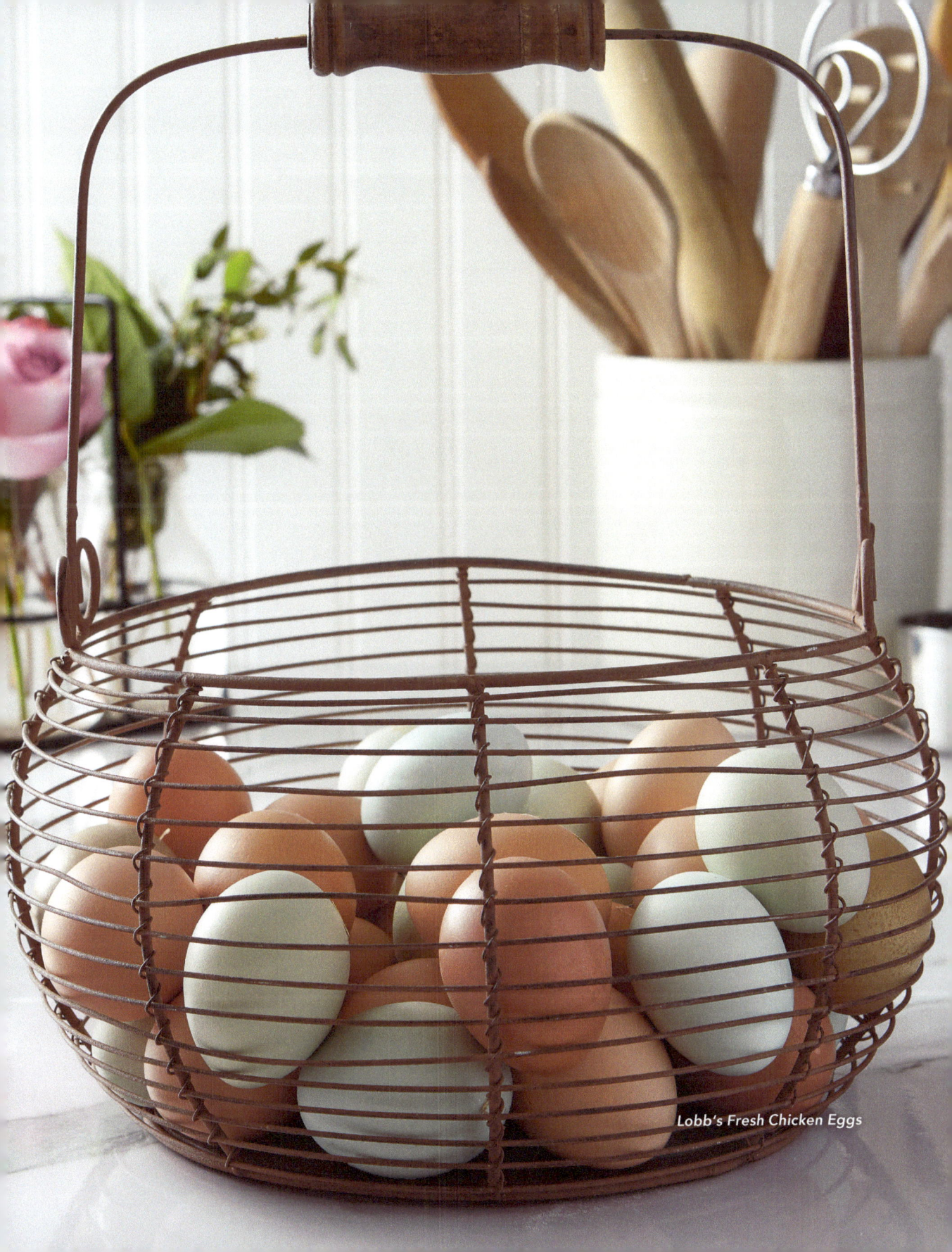

Lobb's Fresh Chicken Eggs

Measuring Techniques

When I teach cooking classes, students are surprised to discover measuring cups for liquid and dry ingredients are different. In most recipes, the difference ends up being negligible. However, in gluten-free sourdough recipes, the differences can add up and affect the outcome.

Liquid ingredients such as water should be measured with liquid measuring cups. Dry ingredients such as flour need to be measured in dry measuring cups according to **How to Measure Flour** instructions. For details on types of measuring cups, see the **Measuring Tools** glossary (p. 101).

How to Measure Flour

Using a scale to weigh ingredients won't be necessary – if you follow these simple steps. While some bakers consider weighing ingredients with a kitchen scale the gold standard, my patients and students have shared for years how the intimidation of using a kitchen scale is a deal breaker to baking at home. By using Imperial measuring cups, we remove that obstacle making it easier to achieve great results in your kitchen.

All recipes in this book were created using the spoon-and-sweep method. Scooping or dipping into flour with measuring cups compacts the flour and increases the measured volume. I refrigerate my preferred gluten-free flour blend, **Bob's Red Mill Gluten-Free 1-to-1 Baking Flour**, in a large airtight container. Stir it with a whisk or Danish dough hook before each use.

Spoon-and-Sweep Method

1. Pour flour into a large bowl or container.

2. Whisk well to eliminate clumps and to aerate.

3. Ladle flour with a spoon into a dry measuring cup until overflowing. Do not pack or tap down flour.

4. Using a flat edge, like the back of a butter knife, sweep to level off excess flour.

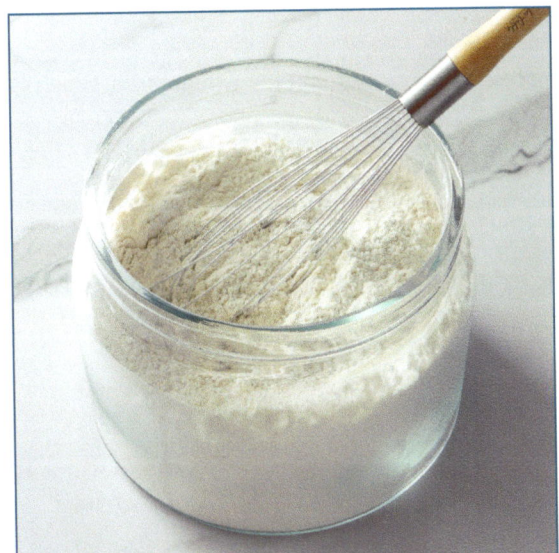

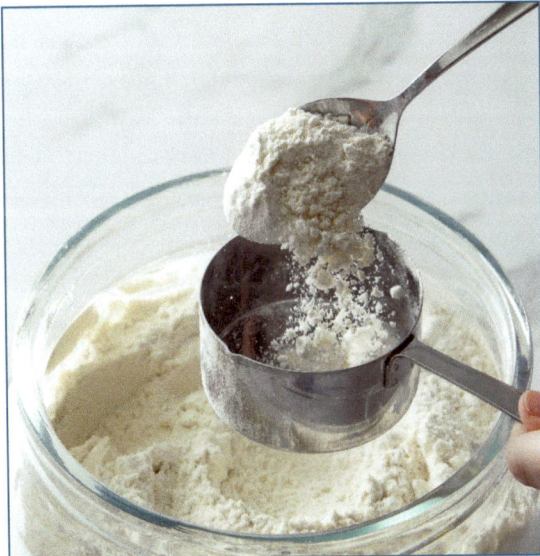

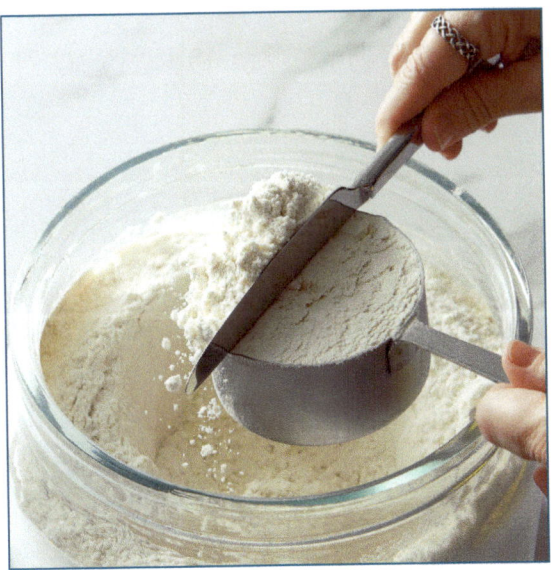

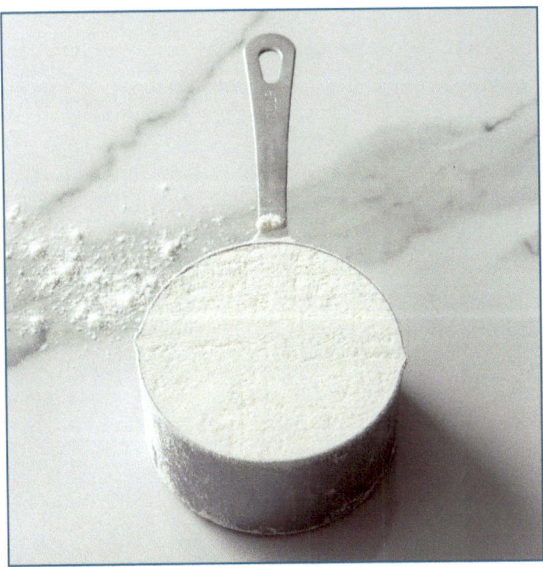

Starter Care

This section is arranged and clearly labeled by subtopic for ease of reference. However, I recommend you read the next four pages in one sitting to get the big picture. It covers everything from how and what to feed your starter to how to store and use it. If questions or issues about your starter come up, look back over this section!

Feeding

Feeding sourdough starter always refers to adding both flour blend and water in equal volume.

Feed with equal parts by volume of gluten-free flour blend and filtered water at regular intervals, typically once a week depending on the use of your starter. Feeding amount depends on recipe use and need for growth. This can range from 1 tablespoon to 1 cup.

To maintain starter volume, feed the same volume discarded. For example, with a recipe calling for 1/2 cup gluten-free sourdough starter, stir your starter then measure 1/2 cup using a dry ingredient measuring cup. Next, feed with 1/2 cup gluten-free flour blend and 1/2 cup water.

Wash hands and all utensils well before each use to minimize chance of unwanted contamination.

Stir with a clean rubber spatula or wooden spoon making sure there are no dry pockets.

The ideal starter consistency is like thick pancake batter.

To encourage your starter to be bubblier and more active, use warm filtered water (85 degrees F) when feeding.

A very warm environment can cause rapid growth that will require more frequent feeding and discarding, for best results, store your starter in the refrigerator.

Only add gluten-free flour and filtered water to your starter, nothing else. On rare occasion, you can sprinkle lightly with dry active yeast granules to increase or stimulate activity.

Discarding

Discard simply refers to removing some starter.

All recipes in this book use discard everywhere *gluten-free sourdough starter* is listed.

Always stir starter and remove desired amount of discard before feeding.

Think of discarding as cleaning house. Healthy, growing yeasts create natural wastes just like when fermenting wine and beer. The tangy sourdough smell we love is the result of a good balance of healthy yeasts and natural byproducts.

Feeding sourdough starter means adding equal volumes of both flour blend and water.

Starter Care (Continued)

Gluten-Free Flour Selection

A gluten-free flour blend is ideal for feeding sourdough starter such as Bob's Red Mill Gluten-Free 1-to-1 Baking Flour Blend, which was used in all recipe testing and development. A blend of gluten-free flours produces a strong starter with consistent baking results. Single-source flour such as brown rice flour or sorghum flour can be used on occasion. Avoid feeding a single-source flour with high starch content like tapioca flour, as they can weaken the starter. See page 104 for more on flour subsitutions.

Water

Use filtered and non-chlorinated water when feeding your gluten-free sourdough starter. Chlorine and other chemicals in tap water can inhibit the growth of beneficial wild yeast and good bacteria in your starter affecting its fermentation activity.

Maintenance

If you have not used or fed your starter for two weeks, discard one-third to one-half then feed. If the consistency gets too thick or thin, simply add a bit more water or flour to adjust. Regularly observe your gluten-free sourdough starter for signs of good fermentation activity, such as bubbles and a tangy smell.

Hooch is the liquid that separates from the solids after a period of yeast activity. Observe the hydration of your starter, if it has been too thick, stir in the hooch, discard and feed. If your starter consistency has gotten too thin, lift or drill a hole along the side of the jar to pour off some of that excess liquid, then discard and feed.

Storage

Keep your gluten-free sourdough starter in a clean, glass container covered with a tidy square of cheesecloth in the back of a refrigerator (40 degrees F).

Freezing

Freeze a 1/2 cup portion sealed in a small glass jar for 6 months at a time. Thaw slowly in the refrigerator and feed daily (1 tablespoon flour and 1 tablespoon water) to reinvigorate.

If your starter gets low on bubbles after freezing, sprinkle with dry active yeast granules then feed in small amounts. If this does not seem to activate your starter, set at room temperature and feed small amounts twice daily for two to three days.

Drying

To dry sourdough starter, spread 1/2 cup in a thin, even layer on rimmed baking sheet lined with a silicone baking mat. Depending on humidity and temperature, drying takes 8 to 12 hours. Starter will lose all gloss and crack when completely dry. Store in airtight container up to 6 months.

Sharing

To divide your starter for sharing, simply save the discard and feed it as a new starter. Alternatively, feed your starter extra amounts until you have enough to divide.

Using

Before using your starter that has not been fed in a week to 10 days, remove some discard, feed, then set at room temperature to encourage yeast activity. The amount of bubbles and a fresh beer smell are indicators for yeast activity. For most recipes, it is not necessary to the bring starter to room temperature before use unless vigorous rise activity is required.

Feed your starter after each use. Typically, the amount fed after each use is equal to the amount used in the recipe. This helps to keep your starter volume consistent.

When vigorous yeast activity is needed, as for the Simple Boule recipe, discard and feed daily until active. A very active starter will almost double in size with bubbles after 6 to 8 hours of feeding, even in the refrigerator.

Starter Troubleshooting Chart

Starter Problem	Solution
Strong odor like a brewery –	nothing wrong, beer-like smell is desirable
Strong odor like vinegar –	discard* then feed
Very strong odor like stinky feet –	probably contaminated, throw away and start over
Graying –	discard* and feed
Pink, orange or charcoal spots –	contaminated, throw away and start over
No bubbles –	discard* and feed frequently to activate
Separation of water from solids –	stir (read more about hooch in Starter Care)
Poor texture, low activity or drab color –	use higher quality flour or reverse osmosis filtered water
Dried flaking starter on sides of jar –	nothing wrong, stir flakes back in as desired

*discard up to half of the total volume

Gluten-Free Sourdough Starter

Making gluten-free sourdough starter or *mother* is easier than you could imagine. You can be up and baking in just about a week. There is no need for complicated instructions or measuring devices. The best way to grow and care for starter is to rely on your eyes and nose. Watch how the bubble formations differ day to day. Pay attention to subtle odor changes, from fresh dough to beer-like yeast.

Be sure to read all of chapter one, especially **Starter Care**, before beginning.
Perform the instructions for feeding your starter about the same time each day.

Equipment
- Sanitized wide-mouth pint or quart-sized jar*
- 7-inch square unbleached cheesecloth
- Wide mouth jar metal ring or rubber band
- Rubber spatula or properly sanitized and oiled wooden spoon
- Imperial measuring cups

*If using pint-sized wide-mouth jar, reduce all flour and water volumes from 1/4 cup to 2 tablespoons

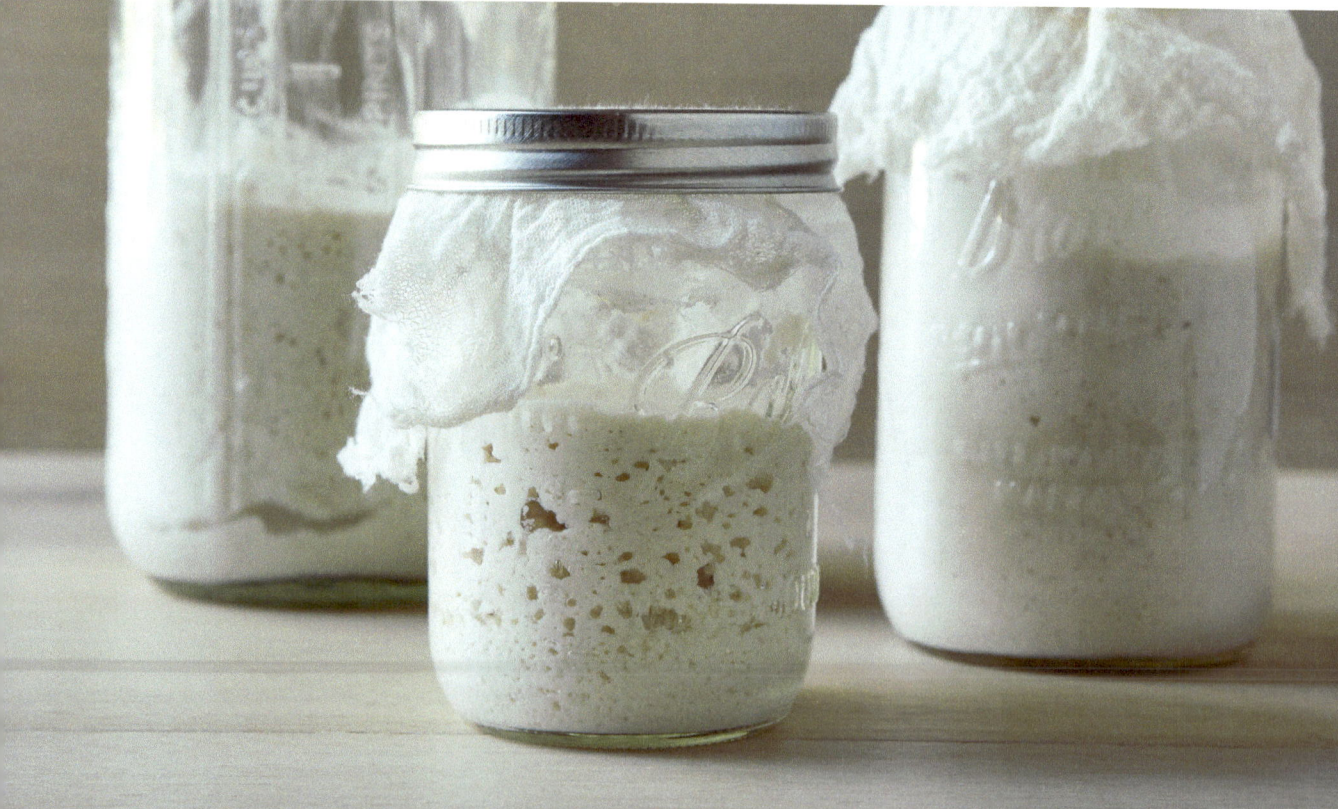

Day 1

Stir 1/4 cup gluten-free flour blend and 1/4 cup water in jar. Secure cheesecloth with metal ring or rubber band. Place in clean, draft-free kitchen area away from direct sunlight.

Day 2

Stir and cover with cheesecloth. Do not add any flour or water today.

Day 3

Add 1/4 cup flour blend and 1/4 cup water. Stir and cover with cheesecloth. Bubbles and slight tangy odor may begin to develop.

Day 4

Stir then discard one-half of the mixture. Add 1/4 cup flour blend and 1/4 cup water. Stir and cover with cheesecloth.

Day 5

Notice bubbles and an earthy, sour smell. Stir then discard one-half of the mixture. Add 1/4 cup flour blend and 1/4 cup water. Stir and cover with cheesecloth.

Day 6

Notice a distinct vinegar or beer smell. Stir then discard one-half of the mixture. Add 1/4 cup flour blend and 1/4 cup water. Stir and cover with cheesecloth.

Day 7

Starter will now have bubbles and a beer-like smell. Stir then discard one-half of the mixture. Add 1/4 cup flour blend and 1/4 cup water. Stir and cover with cheesecloth.

Congratulations! You now have an active starter, known affectionally as *mother*. Store refrigerated and covered with cheesecloth.

To increase the amount of your starter, simply feed daily to reach desired volume, do not remove discard.

Prep time
5 minutes daily for 7 days

Ingredients
Bob's Red Mill Gluten-Free
1-to-1 Baking Flour
Filtered or bottled water

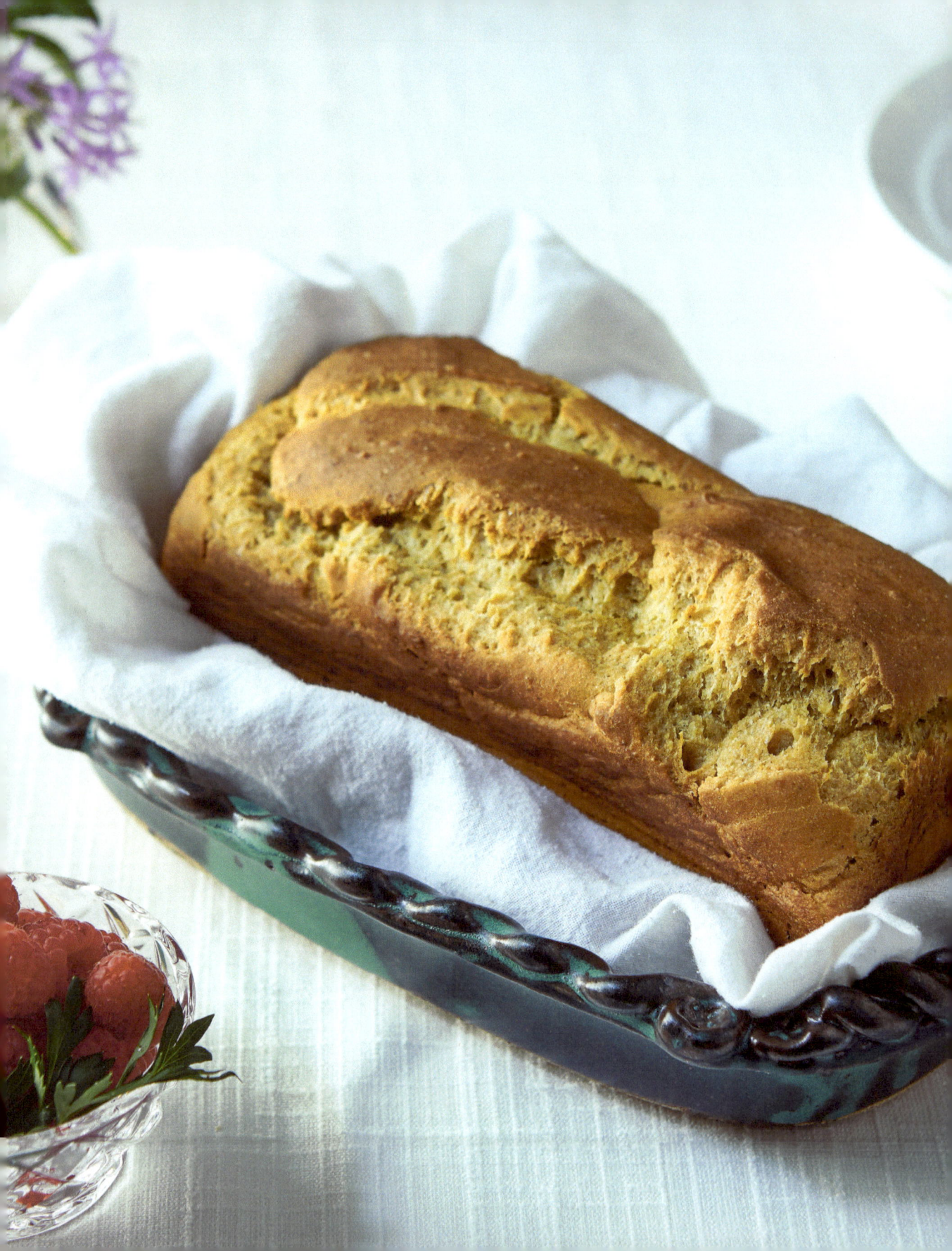

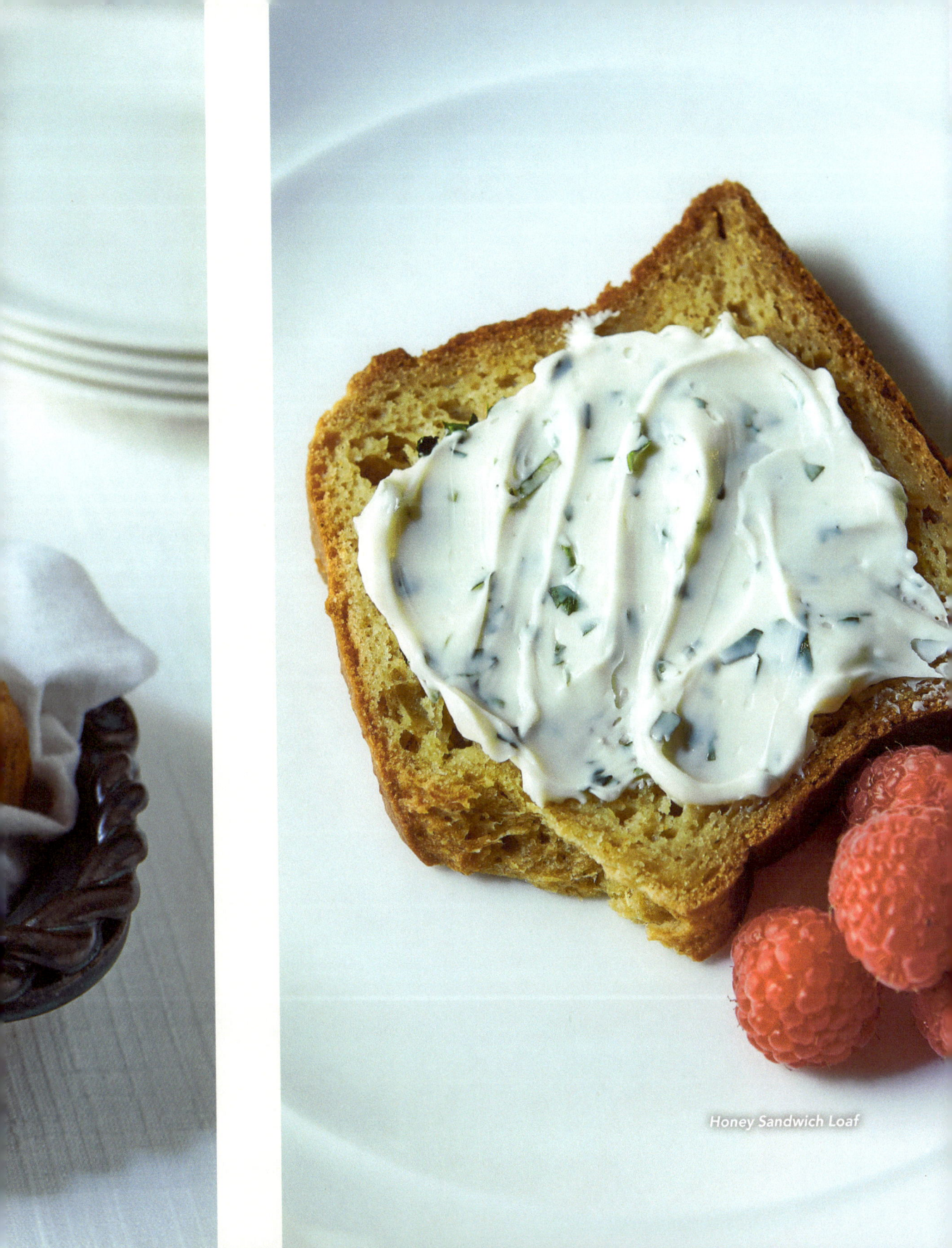

Honey Sandwich Loaf

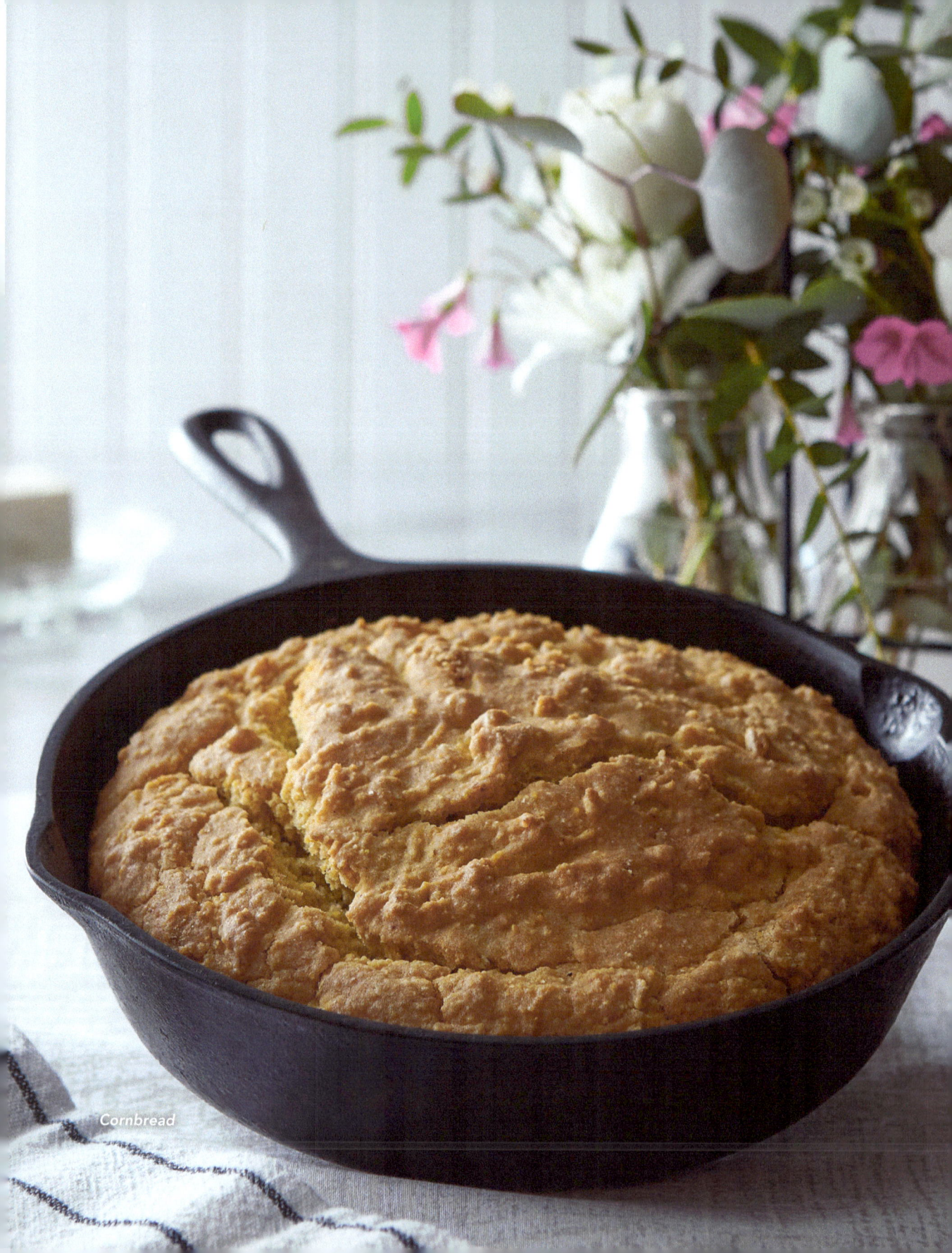

Cornbread

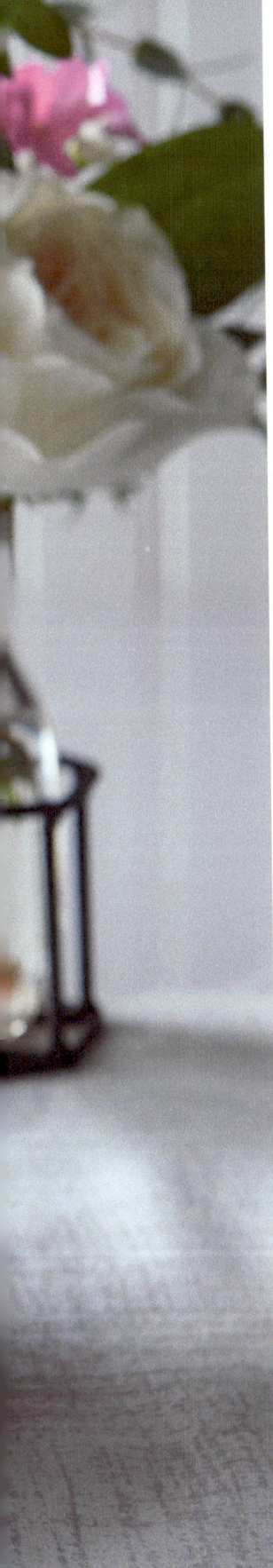

Quick Breads

This chapter is filled with reliable and delicious recipes you are sure to bake often! Some of these recipes use dry active yeast in addition to the sourdough yeast to assist rising. This guarantees great results and without long rise times. Using gluten-free sourdough starter helps keep breads moist and pliable, while imparting that distinctive, subtle and tangy flavor. In this chapter, you'll find good old-fashioned Biscuits, hearty Cornbread, and savory Naan. These easy-to-make recipes will help build confidence in your gluten-free baking skills!

Biscuits

prep time	bake time	yield
20 minutes	**20 minutes**	**4 3-inch biscuits**

My grandmother could whip up a batch of buttermilk biscuits without even reaching for a measuring spoon. Her natural talent in the kitchen created something truly special. Inspired by her legacy, we can also perform a bit of intuitive magic using a dough blade and food processor. These biscuits deliver the salty, buttery goodness I remember. I think Granny would approve!

Equipment: Food processor with dough blade, Bench scraper

1/3 cup milk alternative

1 tablespoon fresh lemon juice

1 cup gluten-free flour blend, plus 1/4 cup for kneading

1/2 cup sorghum flour

1/4 cup brown rice flour

1 tablespoon baking powder

1 teaspoon salt

1/2 teaspoon baking soda

1/2 cup (1 stick) vegan butter, diced and frozen

1/2 cup sourdough starter

In a small bowl, stir together milk and lemon juice. Set aside.

In a food processor with dough blade, whisk flour blend, sorghum flour, rice flour, baking powder, salt and baking soda.

Add frozen butter to flour mixture and pulse to make a crumble (see image p. 97-98). Stop to stir in excess flour from corners. Transfer to medium mixing bowl. If the butter begins to soften, freeze for 10 minutes. Small pieces of frozen butter are key to a fluffy result.

Mix in sourdough starter, milk mixture to butter crumble to form a loose ball.

Working quickly, turn onto flour dusted surface. Use a bench scraper to shape dough into a rectangle. Cut this in half and stack the two pieces. Press gently into another rectangle. Do this process once more leaving the dough in a 2 1/2-inch tall rectangle, or the desired height of biscuits. Wrap with plastic wrap and freeze 30 minutes.

Cut dough into 2-inch squares using a single downward slice, a sawing motion will inhibit the rise. Separate slices 1-inch apart. Cover and freeze for at least 2 hours or up to 1 month in airtight container. Freezing dough maintains loft and shape when baking.

Preheat oven to 425 degrees F. Arrange frozen biscuits 1-inch apart on a rimmed baking sheet lined with baking mat or parchment paper. Bake 20 minutes or until golden brown.

I keep a few diced sticks of vegan butter ready for use in the freezer. Freeze leftover biscuits in airtight container. Reheat in the microwave wrapped in a damp paper towel.

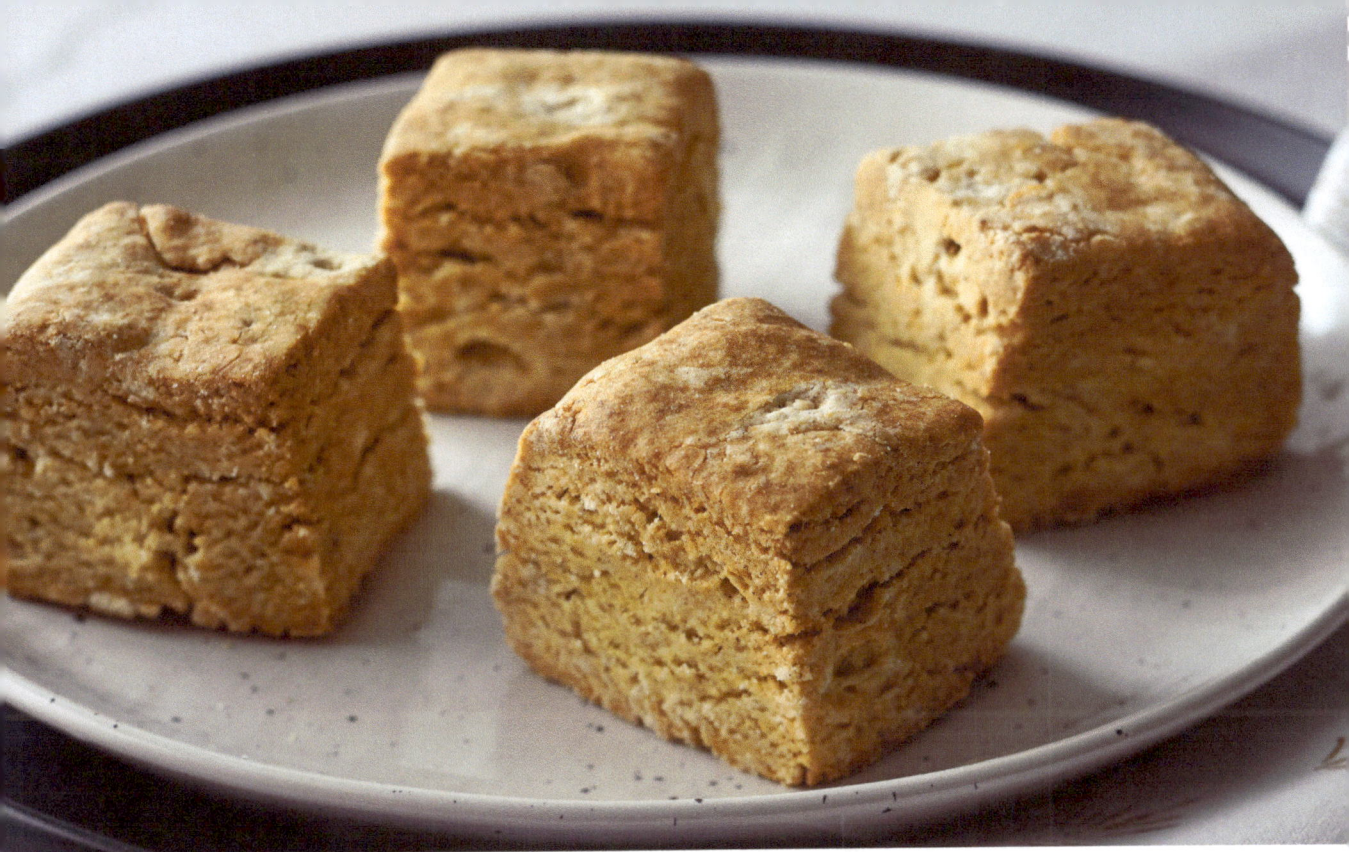

Baking Powder

yield
about 1 cup

Living healthy can sometimes feel like a moving target. So, take baking powder off your worry list! Avoid unwanted ingredients and the possibility of aluminum ingestion by making this large batch at home. Baking powder contains cream of tartar which acts as an activator to release carbon dioxide. Baking soda contributes an alkaline component which helps create the bubbles crucial for rise. The starch binds these ingredients together and regulates the reaction between the acid and alkaline components.

Whisk or sift each ingredient separately before measuring. Use the Spoon-and-Sweep measuring technique over clean parchment to reduce waste.
In a medium bowl, whisk to thoroughly combine. Store in airtight container.

1/2 cup cream of tartar
1/4 cup arrowroot, cornstarch or potato starch
1/4 cup baking soda

Use this baking powder in place of store-bought, measuring it the same.

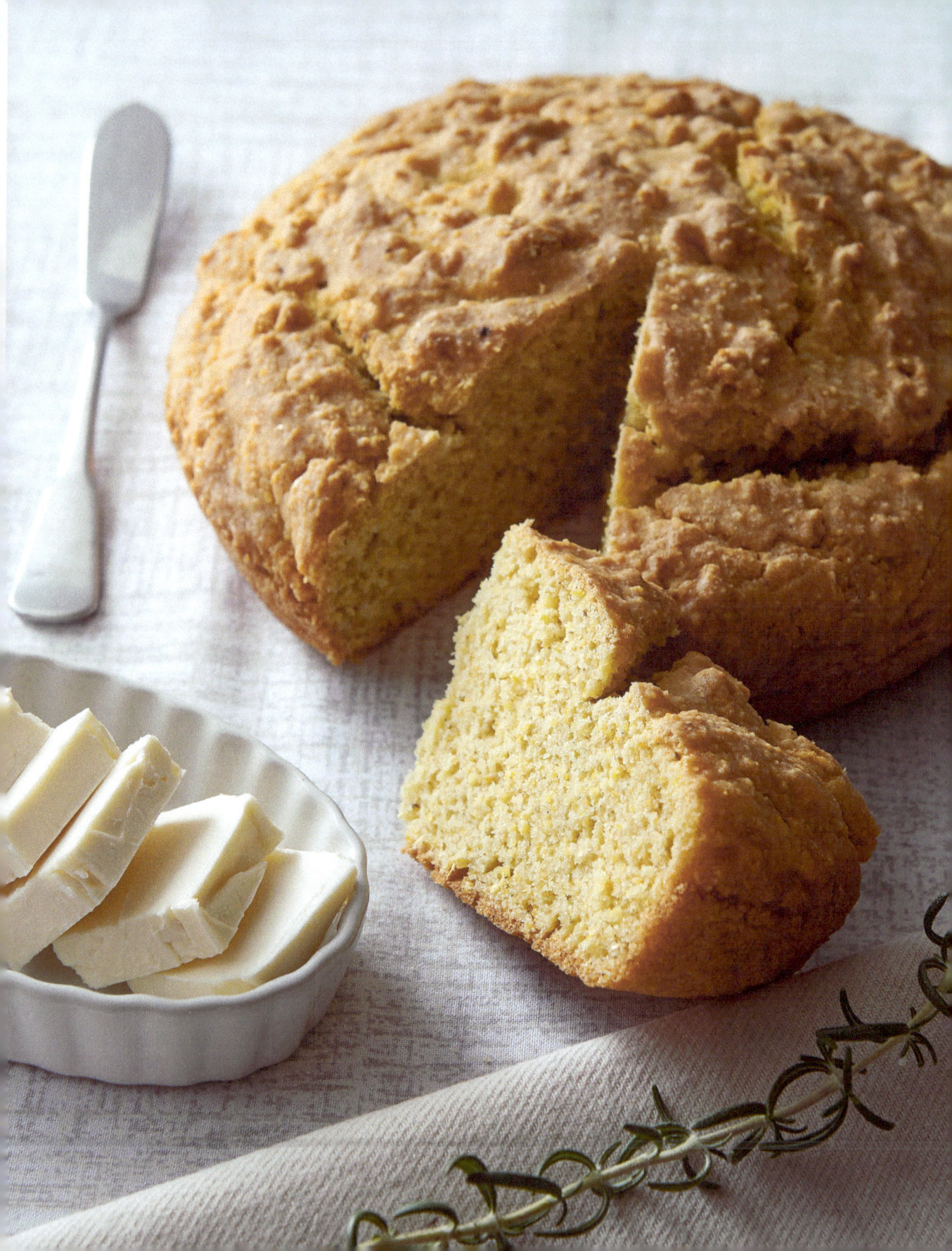

Cornbread

prep time	bake time	yield
5 minutes plus	**30 minutes**	**9 2-inch servings**
30 minutes rest		

My mom used to enjoy a "cornbread shake" – a simple treat made by crumbling leftover cornbread and covering it with milk. We haven't had any leftovers to make a shake with this recipe yet, though! This gluten-free cornbread bakes up beautifully golden and makes a perfect side for beans, chili, stews and more. Cornmeal is often at risk of cross-contact with wheat during manufacturing, so be sure to choose gluten-free cornmeal depending on your needs. Use stone ground cornmeal for an old-fashioned texture.

In a medium bowl, whisk cornmeal, flour blend, baking powder, sugar and salt.

Add starter, eggs, melted butter and milk. Whisk to thoroughly combine. Set aside to rest for 30 minutes.

Preheat oven to 400 degrees F. Generously butter 8-by-8-inch glass baking dish or melt 1 tablespoon butter or olive oil in a hot 7-inch cast iron skillet. Spread batter in prepared dish.

Bake 30 minutes or until golden brown. Serve warm.

1 cup cornmeal
2/3 cup gluten-free flour blend
1 tablespoon baking powder
1 tablespoon sugar
1 teaspoon salt

1 cup gluten-free sourdough starter
2 eggs, beaten
4 tablespoons vegan butter, melted plus more for pan
1/4 cup milk alternative

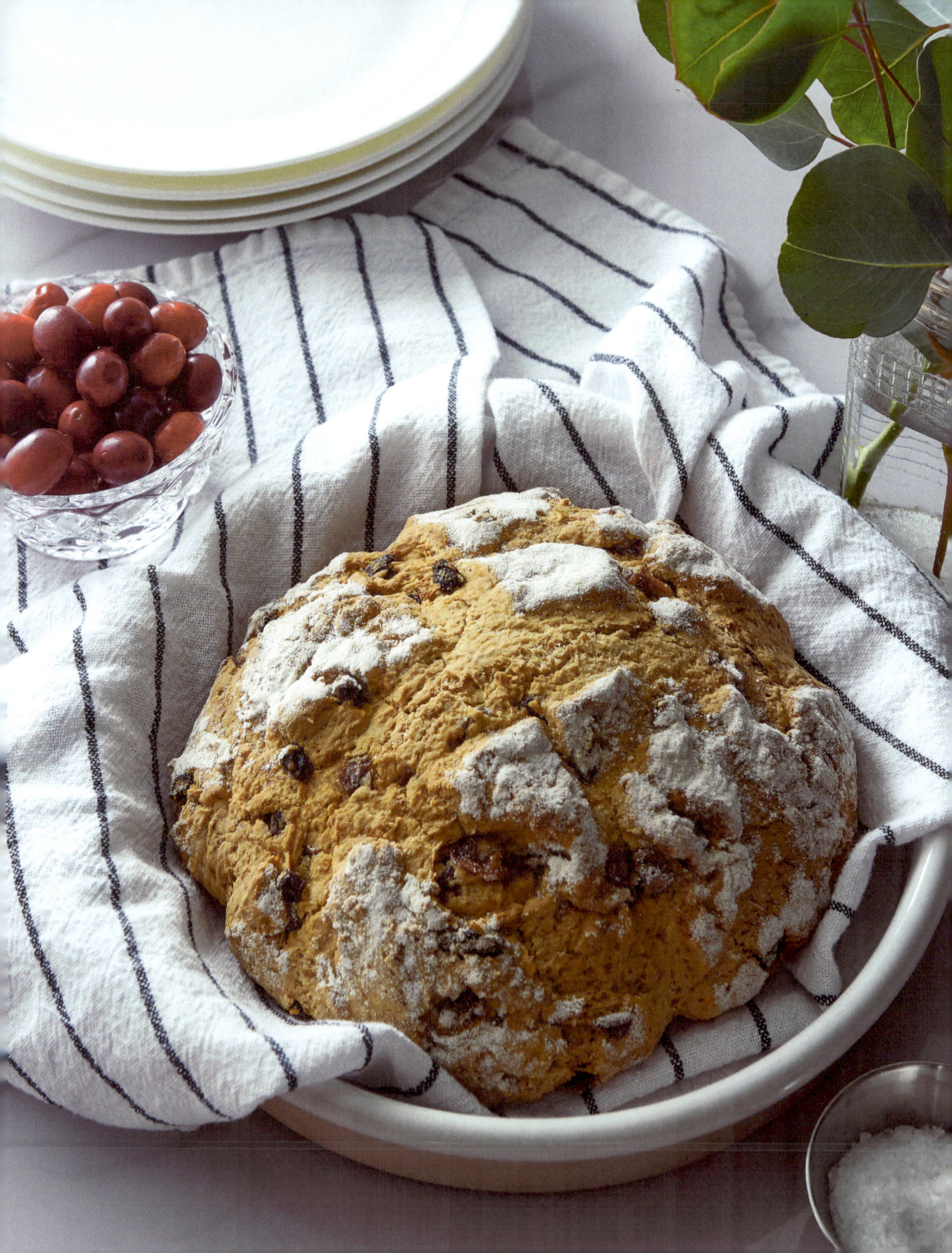

Irish Soda Bread

prep time	bake time	yield
15 minutes plus 4 hours chill	**60 minutes**	**7-inch round loaf**

Inspired by soda bread I enjoyed in Ireland years ago, this recipe aims to be more traditional versus some modern versions containing excess baking soda which can make the bread dark and taste of soda. This is an easy bread to make but it has a short shelf life. According to Irish folklore, be sure to cut the traditional 'X' across the top to let out the fairies!

Equipment: Stand mixer with dough hook attachment

Lightly oil loaf pan. In a small bowl, combine milk and lemon juice. Set aside.

1/2 cup milk alternative
1 tablespoon fresh lemon juice

In a stand mixer with dough hook attachment, whisk flour blend, sorghum flour, potato starch, psyllium, sugar, baking powder, baking soda and salt. Add starter, milk mixture and egg to flour mixture. Mix on low to combine. Scrape clean the sides and bottom of the bowl with a rubber spatula. Mix on medium for 3 minutes more. Mix in dried fruit if using. Dough will be sticky. Transfer to a lightly oiled small bowl. The loaf will take the size and shape of this bowl. Cover and refrigerate at least 4 hours. Baking cold dough maintains its shape.

1 cup gluten-free flour blend
1/2 cup sorghum or millet flour
1/2 cup potato starch or tapioca starch
1 tablespoon psyllium husk fiber
1 tablespoon sugar
2 teaspoons baking powder
1 teaspoon baking soda
1/2 teaspoon salt

Preheat oven to 375 degrees F.

Invert dough and place on baking mat or parchment lined baking sheet. Dust with flour blend or brown rice flour and cut a 1/2-inch deep 'X' across the top and sides.

1/2 cup gluten-free sourdough starter
1 egg, beaten

Bake 45 minutes or until crust reaches deep golden brown. Loosely tent with foil if crust browns before internal temperature reaches 210 degrees F. Cool completely on a wire rack before slicing.

Variations
Spotted Dog
Add 1/2 cup raisins or dried cranberries rehydrated in hot water for 10 minutes and drained, making what the Irish call Spotted Dog or Railway Cake.

Naan

prep time	bake time	yield
10 minutes	**6 to 8 minutes per naan**	**6 flatbreads (6-by-8-inch oval)**

Like many Texans, I often want a tortilla with virtually any meal. This gluten-free sourdough naan bread is a wonderfully soft and pliable substitute. You can easily prepare two dozen in advance and freeze them for later use without sacrificing quality.

Equipment: Rolling pin

1/2 cup coconut flour

1/4 cup almond flour

2 tablespoons psyllium husk fiber

2 teaspoons minced fresh rosemary

1 teaspoon baking powder

1 teaspoon garlic powder

1 teaspoon salt

1/4 cup gluten-free sourdough starter

3 tablespoons melted vegan butter

1 cup boiling water

In a medium bowl, whisk coconut flour, almond flour, psyllium, rosemary, baking powder, garlic powder and salt. Add sourdough starter and butter. Combine with a Danish dough hook or wooden spoon. Mixture will resemble small crumbles.

Add boiling water, stir carefully to form a dough. Divide into 6 even balls.

Between two sheets of parchment paper, roll into ovals about 1/8-inch thick.

Cook on medium-high skillet about 4 minutes on each side until a deep golden. Naan may puff slightly while cooking. Wrap in clean kitchen towel, serve warm.

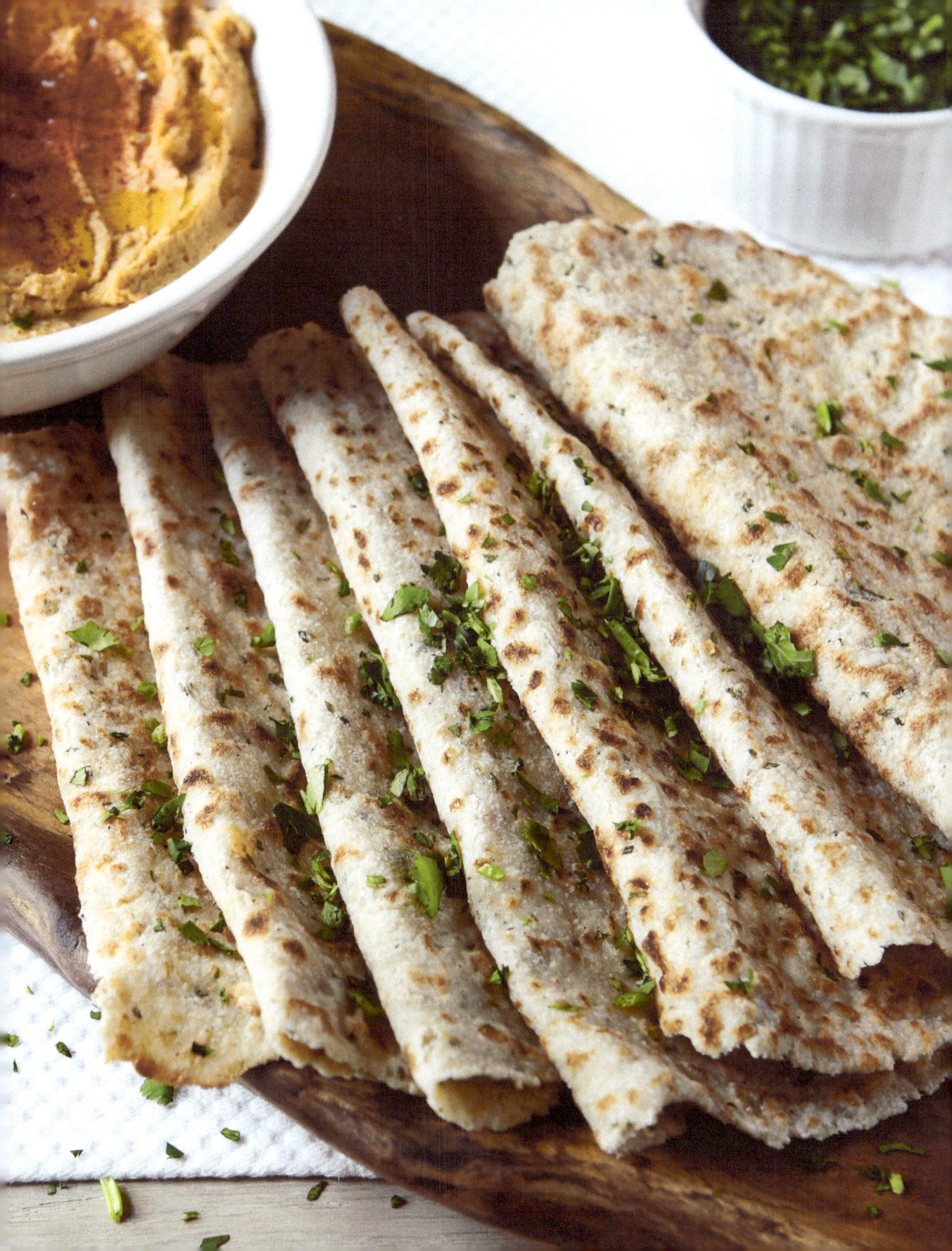

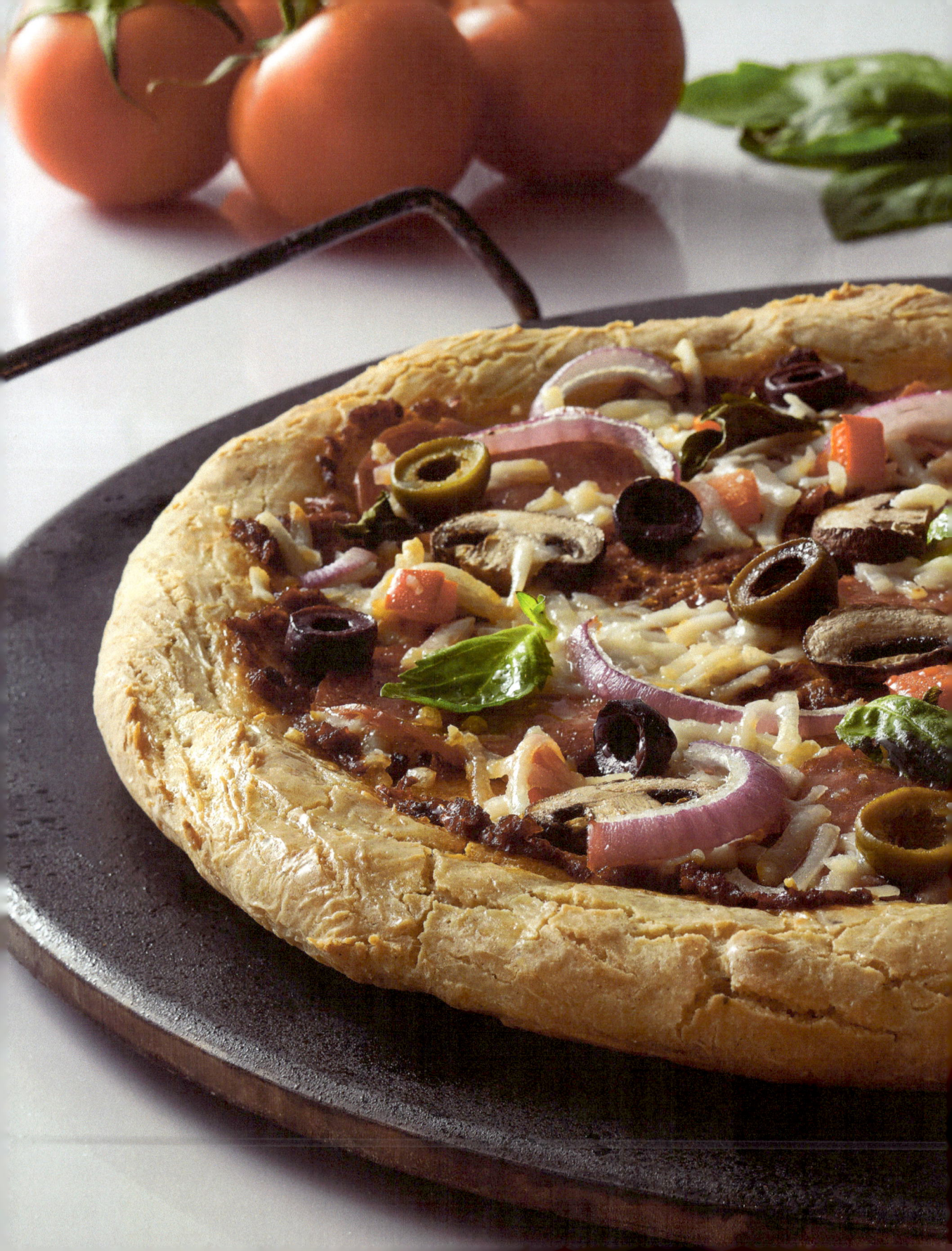

Pizza Crust

prep time	bake time	yield
30 minutes plus	**30 minutes**	**9-by-13-inch crust**
1 hour rise		

Hallelujah! Pizza night is back on the menu! With a crispy crust and soft center, this flavorful gluten-free crust saves your Friday nights. Say goodbye to missed pizza parties and hello to a new family favorite! Don't worry about making too many, this gluten-free crust reheats well, so you can enjoy your delicious creation Saturday morning!

Equipment: Stand mixer with dough hook attachment

Lightly oil a medium baking sheet lined with a baking mat or use a baking stone.

In a stand mixer bowl with a dough hook attachment, whisk flour blend, sorghum flour, psyllium husk, sugar, Italian seasoning, yeast, garlic powder and salt.

To the flour mixture, add warm water, olive oil, starter and apple cider vinegar. Combine on low for 1 minute. Scrape clean the sides and bottom of the bowl with a rubber spatula. Mix on medium for 2 minutes more. Dough will be sticky.

Turn out the dough on the prepared pan and pat gently into desired shape with oiled fingertips.

Cover loosely with plastic wrap and let rise in a draft free place 30 to 60 minutes. Dough will slightly increase in size.

Preheat oven to 450 degrees F with top rack in upper half of oven.

Poke several holes with a fork in the middle to keep dough from bubbling up. Pre-bake 10 minutes.

Arrange your favorite pizza toppings: tomato pesto, uncured pepperoni, diced bell peppers, fresh mushroom slices, oregano and vegan cheese.

Bake 20 minutes or until deep golden brown.

2 cups gluten-free flour blend

2/3 cup sorghum flour

1 tablespoon psyllium husk fiber

1 tablespoon sugar

2 teaspoons dry Italian seasoning

1 teaspoon active dry yeast

1/2 teaspoon garlic powder

1/2 teaspoon sea salt

1 cup warm water (105 to 115 degrees F)

1/4 cup extra virgin olive oil

1/4 cup gluten-free sourdough starter

1 tablespoon apple cider vinegar

Favorite pizza toppings

Pumpkin Bread

prep time	bake time	yield
10 minutes	**90 minutes**	**9-by-5-inch loaf**

Every autumn, I used to be jealous of people eating sweet and rich slices of pumpkin bread at a certain local coffee shop. But not anymore! With the convenience of canned pumpkin puree, this bread is a nutritious delight to be enjoyed year-round. Get creative with add-ins to suit your cravings – whether gooey chocolate chips or crunchy walnuts, you can't go wrong with this simple recipe!

Equipment: Stand mixer with whisk attachment

1/2 cup (1 stick) vegan butter
2/3 cup packed brown sugar

1 1/2 cups (one 14-ounce can) pumpkin puree
1/2 cup milk alternative
1/4 cup gluten-free sourdough starter
3 large eggs
1/2 teaspoon vanilla (optional)

2 cups gluten-free flour blend
1/2 cup almond flour
2 tablespoons baking powder
1 tablespoon pumpkin pie spice
2 teaspoons cinnamon
2 teaspoon baking soda
1/2 teaspoon sea salt

Preheat oven to 350 degrees F. Lightly oil pan.

In a stand mixer with whisk attachment, cream butter and sugar until thoroughly combined.

Add pumpkin, milk, starter, eggs and vanilla if using. Mix on low to combine. Scrape clean sides of the bowl. Mix again on low to medium speed to ensure all liquid ingredients are light in color and slightly fluffy, about 2 minutes.

In a separate medium bowl, whisk flour blend, almond flour, baking powder, pumpkin pie spice, cinnamon, baking soda and sea salt.

Add flour mixture to pumpkin mixture and mix on low until combined. Scrape clean the sides of the bowl with a rubber spatula as needed. Pour into prepared pan.

Bake 90 minutes or until crust is a deep golden brown. Loosely tent with foil if crust browns before internal temperature reaches 210 degrees F. Remove from pan. Cool completely on a wire rack before slicing.

Pumpkin Pie Spice

3 tablespoons Ceylon cinnamon

2 teaspoons ground ginger

2 teaspoons ground nutmeg

1 teaspoon ground allspice

1 teaspoon ground clove

Whisk all spices in a medium bowl. Store in airtight container.

> ### *Variations*
> Add one of these combination of fillings to the batter.
>
> 1/4 to 1/2 cup chopped pecans
>
> 1/4 cup chocolate chips
>
> 1/2 cup chopped walnuts
>
> 1/4 cup dried fruit (raisins, dates or dried cranberries)
>
> 2 tablespoons of pumpkin seeds (pepitas)

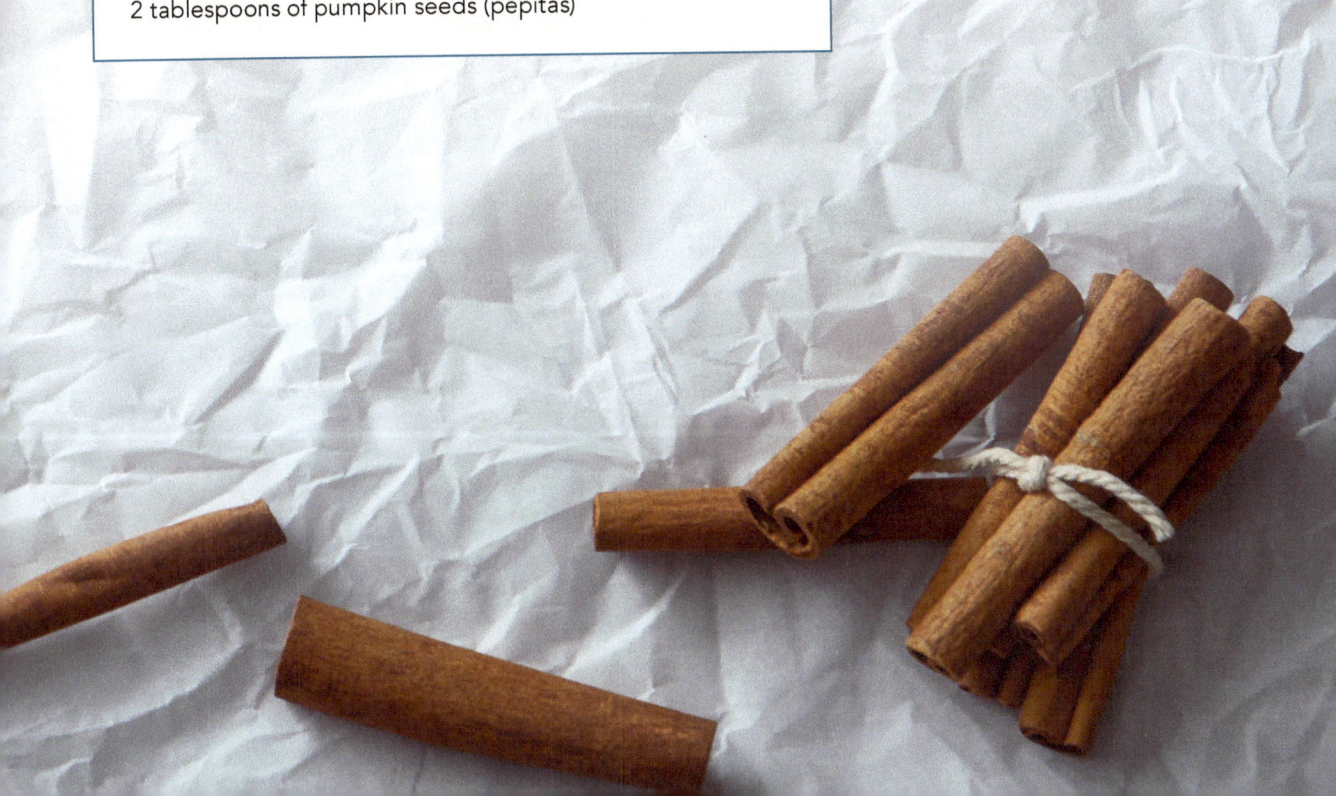

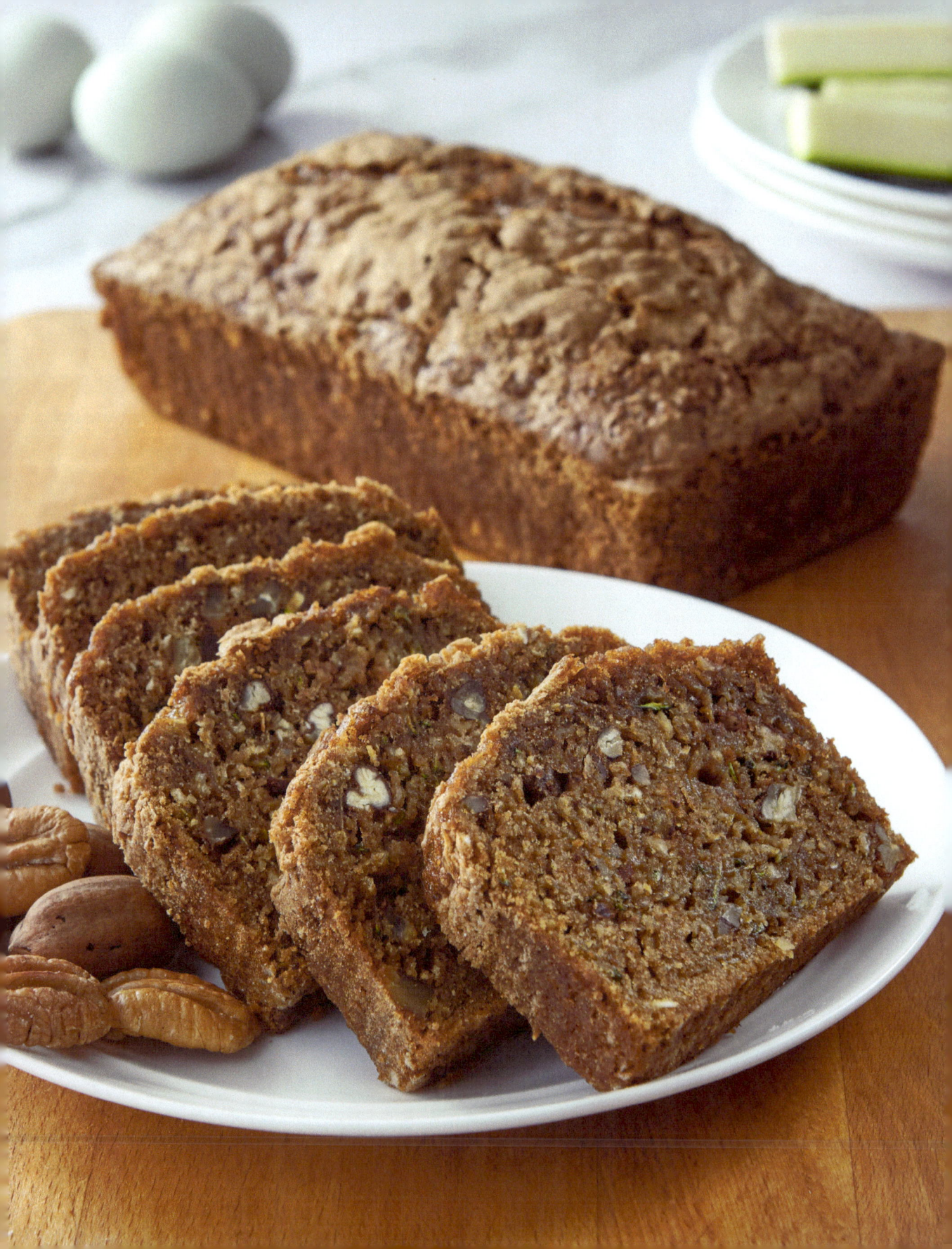

Zucchini Bread

prep time	bake time	yield
10 minutes	**60 minutes**	**9-by-4-inch Pullman loaf**

Ah, nothing holds sweet nostalgia like mom's kitchen! My mom could have mixed her popular zucchini bread with her eyes closed. She made the most delightful, moist loaf that filled our home with warmth and love. After countless attempts to recreate that comforting, rich flavor, I've achieved it with this gluten-free, lower-sugar version. Each slice is like a cinnamon hug. Perfect with a cup of coffee and a sweet memory.

Equipment: Stand mixer with whisk attachment

Preheat oven to 350 degrees F. Lightly oil and flour pan.

In a stand mixer with paddle attachment, beat eggs, sugar and brown sugar. Add oil, starter and vanilla. Mix to thoroughly combine. Scape clean sides of the bowl. Mix again on low speed to ensure all liquid ingredients are combined, about 2 minutes

Add flour blend, oats, cinnamon, baking powder, baking soda and salt. Mix well to combine.

Stir in zucchini and nuts. Pour into prepared pan.

Bake 60 minutes or until crust is dark golden brown. Loosely tent with foil if crust browns before internal temperature reaches 210 degrees F. Remove from pan. Cool completely on wire rack before slicing. Store in airtight container.

2 eggs

1/2 cup sugar

1/2 cup brown sugar

1/4 cup avocado oil or extra virgin oil

1/4 cup gluten-free sourdough starter

2 teaspoons vanilla

1 cup gluten-free flour blend, plus more for dusting loaf pan

1/2 cup quick cooking gluten-free oats (use rolled oats* for a more rustic loaf)

2 teaspoons cinnamon

1/2 teaspoon baking powder

1/2 teaspoon baking soda

1/2 teaspoon salt

1 cup grated zucchini

1/2 cup chopped pecans or walnuts

*I prefer One Degree Organics' Gluten-Free Sprouted Rolled Oats.

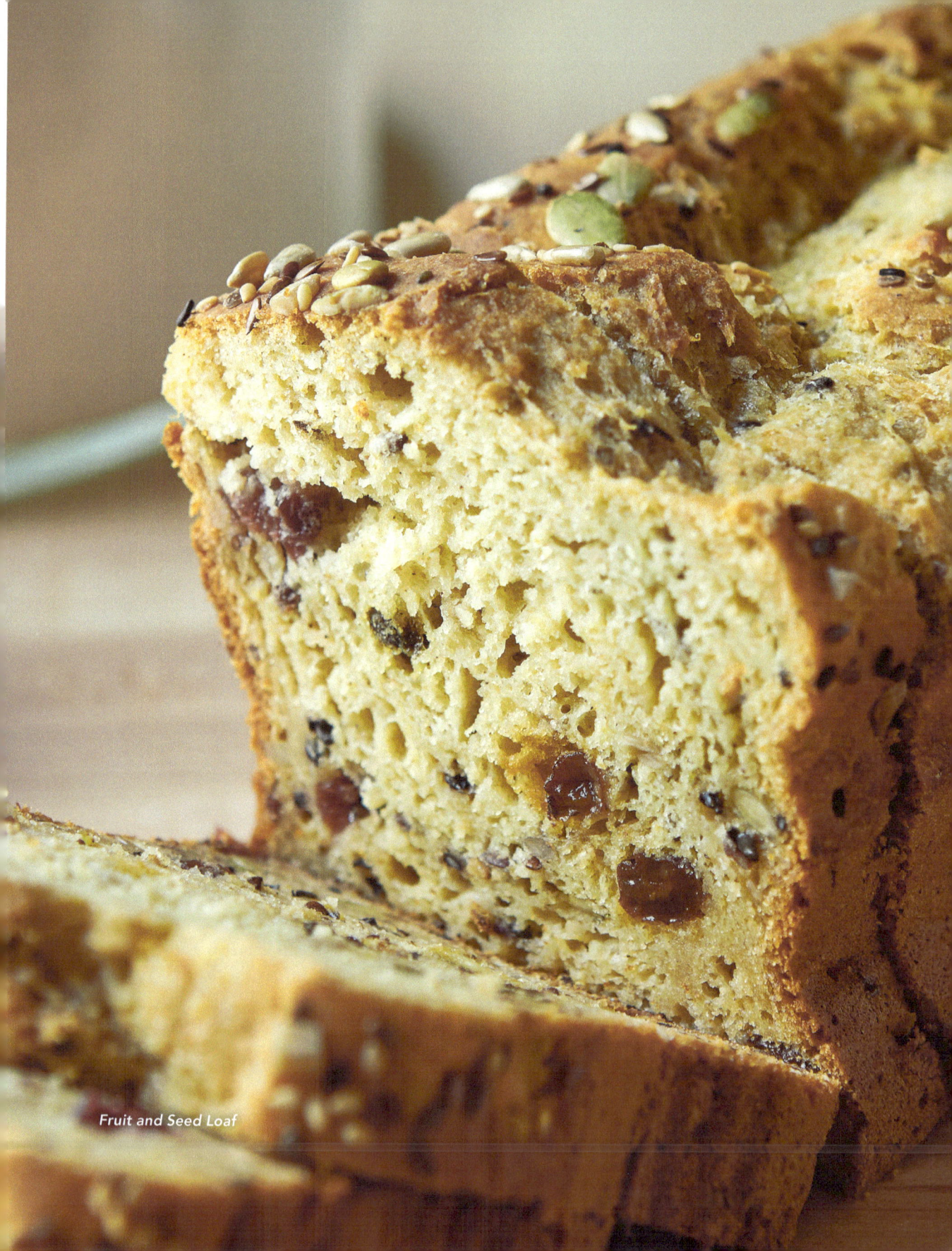

Fruit and Seed Loaf

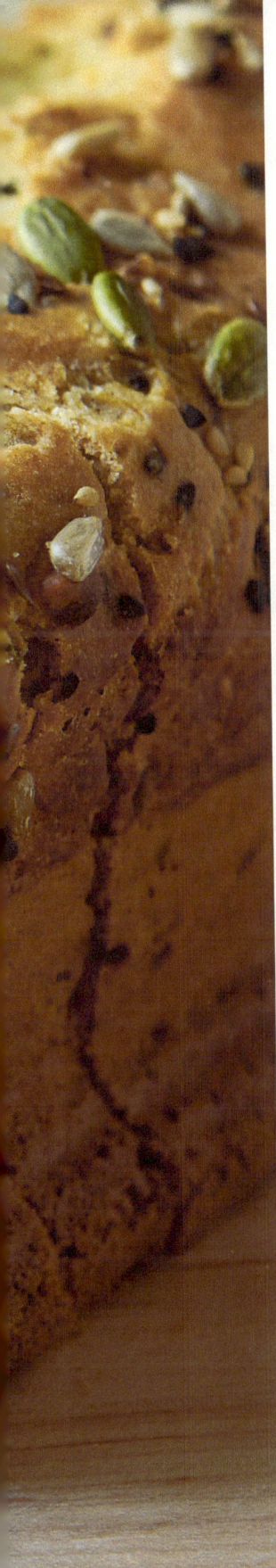

Slow-rise Breads

Some breads just need more time to achieve the desirable rise. I like to reverse engineer the timing for these breads, subtracting cooling, baking, rise and preparation time from when I want the bread to be ready. Perfecting the timing takes practice, but with these recipes, you are sure to end up with delicious bread. Be sure you review the **Get Started** chapter before diving in.

Rising or proofing the dough is best done in a warm (80 degrees F), draft-free place like a warming drawer or oven. To proof in an oven, turn it on for just a few moments to warm, then turn it off. Place the dough near the light and close the door, leave the oven light on. For added warmth, place a pan of hot water on the bottom of the oven, reheating the water as needed.

All the recipes in this chapter need a very active starter, one that increases in size with many bubbles within an hour of feeding. However, if I don't have the time to carefully nuture my starter for several days to be gloriously vigorous – I just add 1 teaspoon of active dry yeast to the dry ingredients and watch the bread rise more quickly!

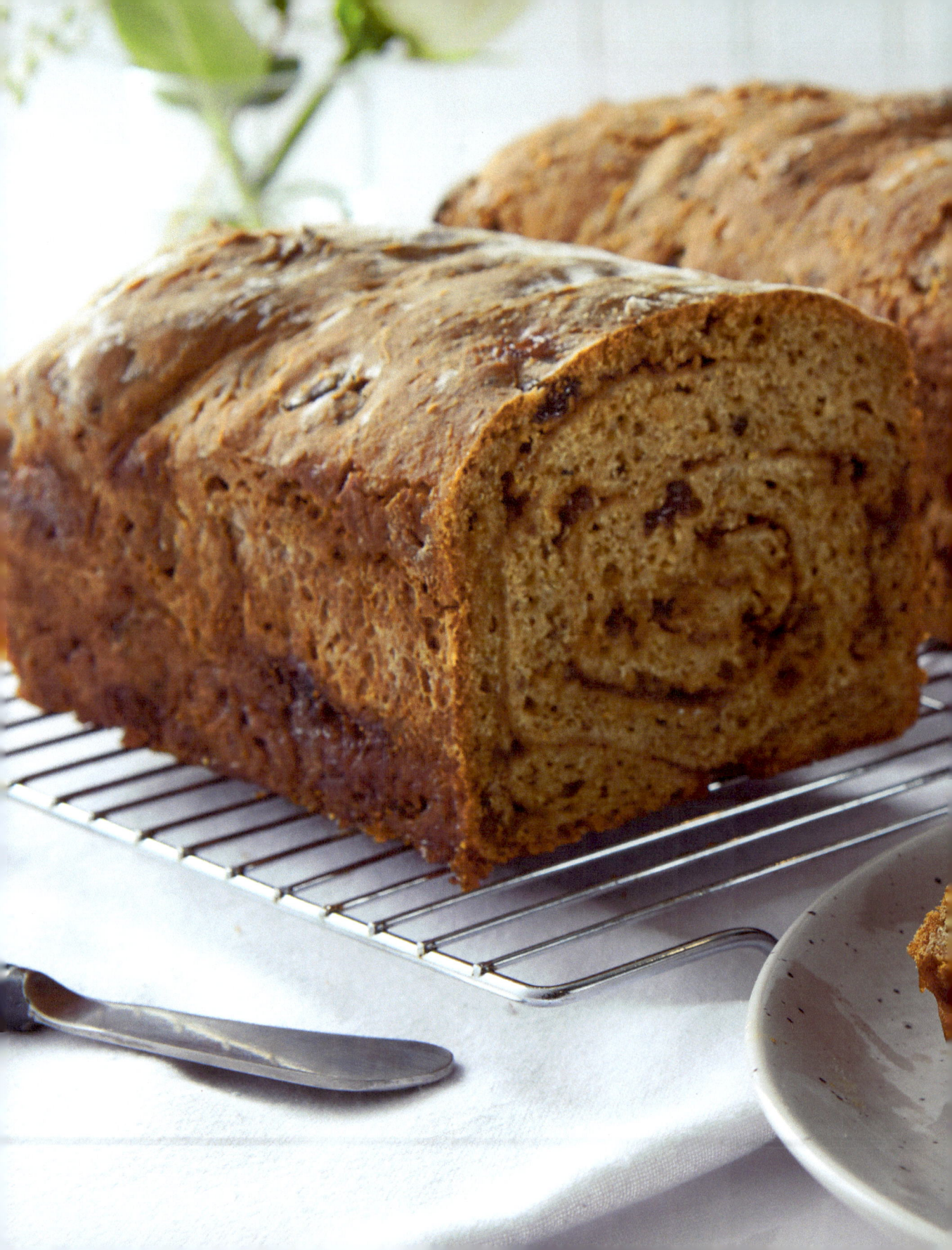

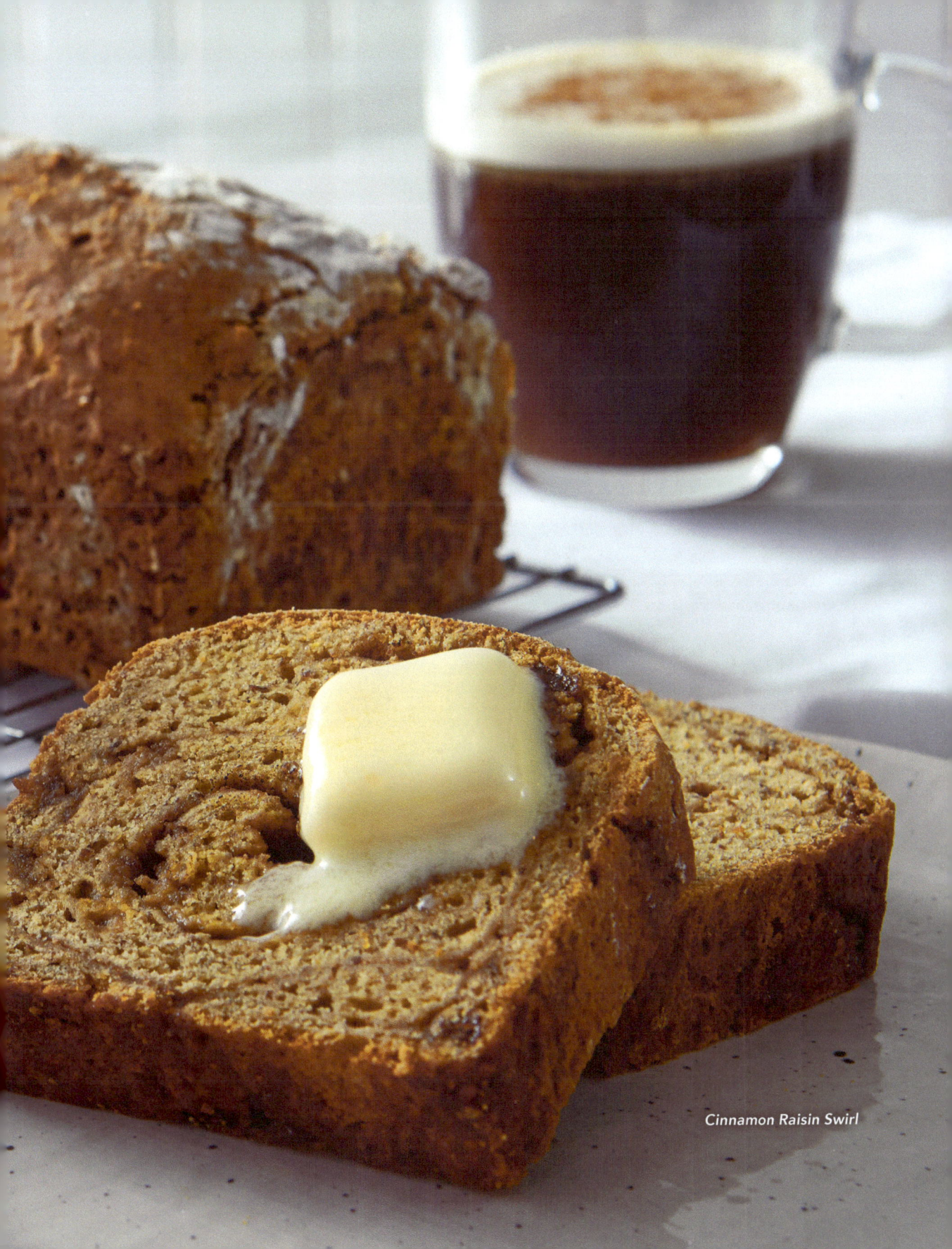

Cinnamon Raisin Swirl

Cinnamon Raisin Swirl

prep time	bake time	yield
15 minutes plus	**60 minutes**	**9-by-4-inch Pullman loaf pan**
2 hours chill and rise		

A favorite in my family, this bread is a cinnamon-sweet variation of the honey sandwich loaf. With the help of active yeast, you'll get a reliable rise perfect whether you are a sourdough baking beginner or just in a hurry. That subtle tangy flavor of the sourdough starter ensures this bread is delicious, moist and elastic without being gummy. Try subsituting raisins with mini chocolate chips. Get ready to bake your new craving!

Equipment: Stand mixer with paddle attachment, Rolling pin

Proof yeast

1 cup warm water (105 to 115 degrees F)

2 tablespoons sugar

1 teaspoon active dry yeast

2 eggs

1/3 cup gluten-free sourdough starter

1/4 cup extra virgin olive oil, plus more to coat pan

1 tablespoon apple cider vinegar

Lightly oil pan. In small glass bowl, stir to dissolve sugar in warm water. Gently stir in yeast. Set aside for 10 minutes. A foam should appear on top.

In medium bowl, whisk flour blend, sorghum flour, ground flax, nutritional yeast, psyllium fiber, baking powder, sugar, cinnamon and salt.

In a stand mixer bowl with paddle attachment, add eggs, sourdough starter, olive oil and apple cider vinegar. Mix on medium speed until egg look combined, but do not whip whites. Add proofed yeast mixture. Mix on low to combine.

Add flour mixture and combine on low speed for 30 seconds to incorporate. Scrape clean sides and bottom of the bowl with a rubber spatula. Mix again on medium for 3 minutes. The batter will be thick and sticky. Stir in raisins. Cover and refrigerate 60 minutes.

Gluten-free breads rely on the sides of the pan to help support the crust.

In a small bowl, combine brown sugar, almond flour and cinnamon. With a rubber spatula, scape dough onto large sheet of plastic wrap or Bee's Wrap dusted with potato starch. Layer another large sheet of plastic wrap on top. Roll into 1/2-inch-thick rectangle about 9- by-20-inches. Carefully remove top sheet of plastic and sprinkle generously with filling mixture leaving a 2-inch border on one short edge to seal. Lift short end of plastic to roll up into a log. If dough sticks to plastic, sprinkle with potato starch and scape using a small rubber spatula. Refrigerate 30 to 60 minutes while working if dough gets too sticky. Gently set in prepared pan with seam side down. Cover with clean dish towel and set aside to rise. Rise time depends on yeast activity and ambient temperature, 30 to 60 minutes. Do not allow the edges of the dough to rise closer than 3/4-inch from the lip of the pan, more rise occurs during baking.

Preheat oven to 375 degrees F with rack arranged in the lower third. Bake 30 minutes. Loosely tent with foil when crust begins to brown. Bake an additional 30 minutes or until internal temperature reaches 210 degrees F.

Cool 20 minutes. Remove from pan. Cool completely on a wire rack before slicing. Bread will lose loft and dry out if sliced while warm.

Flour mixture

2 cups gluten-free flour blend

1 cup sorghum flour

3 tablespoons ground flax seed

2 tablespoons nutritional yeast, flaked

2 tablespoons psyllium husk fiber

2 tablespoons baking powder

2 tablespoons sugar

2 teaspoons cinnamon

1 teaspoon salt

1/2 cup raisins, rehydrated in hot water 10 minutes, drained

Filling

1/3 cup brown sugar

1 tablespoon almond flour

1 tablespoon cinnamon

2 tablespoons potato starch, for dusting

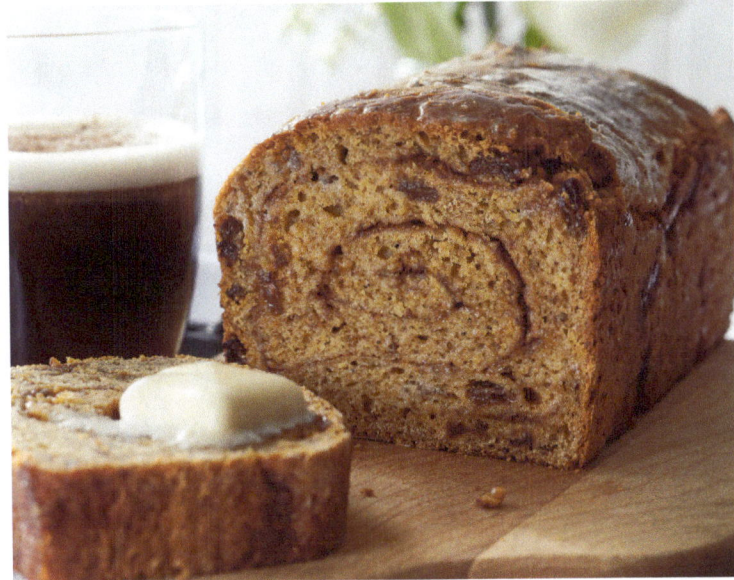

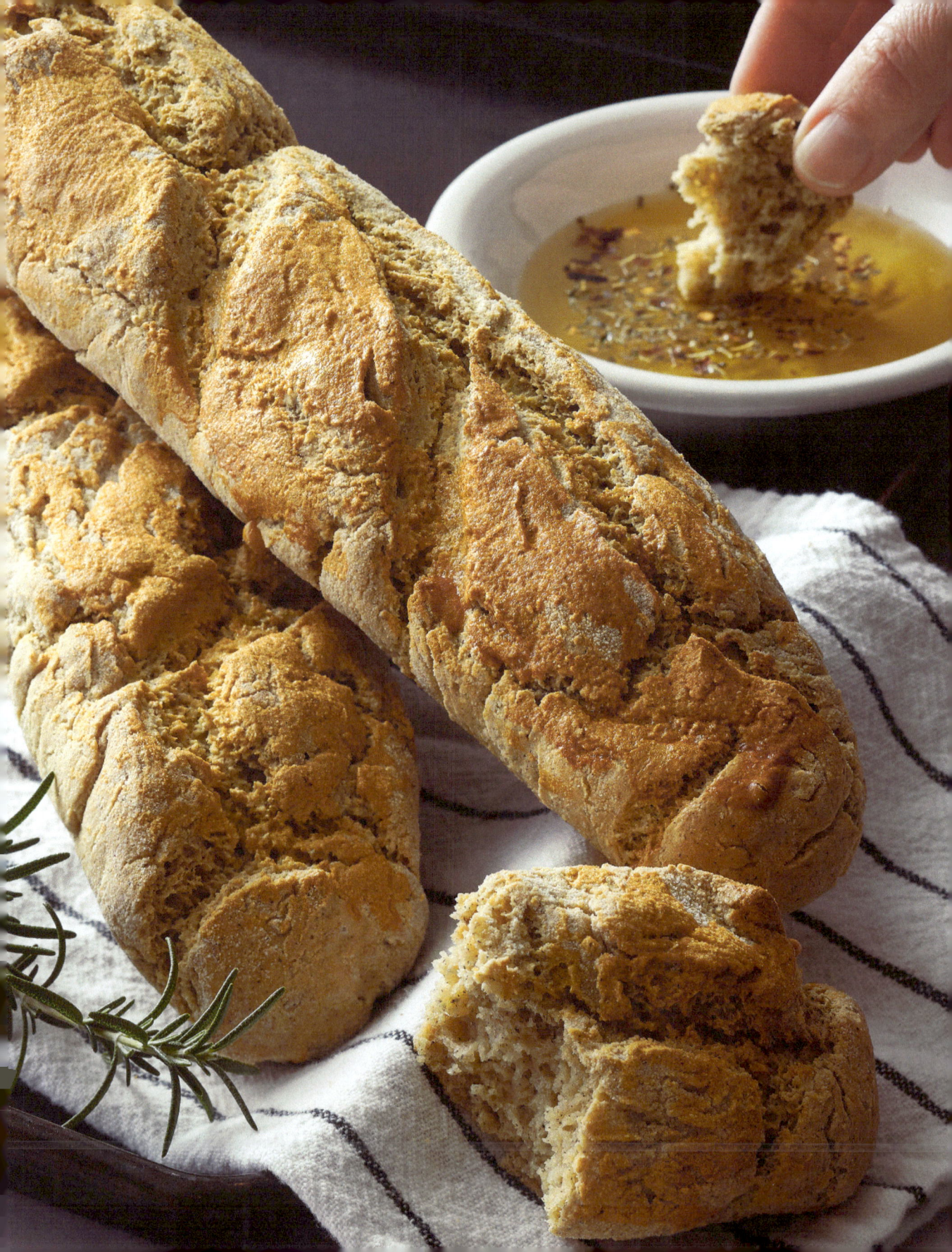

Rustic Baguette

prep time	bake time	yield
10 minutes plus	**30 minutes**	**2 18-inch or 4 demi-loaves**
1 hour 15 minutes rise		

January 2020, right before the pandemic spread across America, I got together with a French baker to make gluten-free baguettes! This is a rustic and sourdough variation inspired by her traditional version with only flour, salt and yeast. Plan ahead, this dough needs to be cold before formed into loaves.

Equipment: Danish dough hook or sturdy rubber spatula, Baguette baking pan (optional)

In a small bowl, combine water, sugar and yeast. Set aside for 10 minutes. A foam should appear on top.

In a small bowl, mix flax seed in olive oil. Set aside.

In a large bowl, whisk flour blend, buckwheat flour and salt. Add yeast mixture, flax mixture, starter and eggs. Stir until a dough forms. The mixture may look like large crumbles then will come together with continued stirring. Cover and refrigerate 60 minutes to hydrate the flours. Dough may increase in size.

Dust a large sheet of parchment paper or a clean linen towel and the dough with buckwheat flour. Evenly divide and shape dough into 2 18-inch or 4 demi-loaves. Make three diagonal slashes 1/2-inch deep across the top. This baguette dough can spread when rising resulting in a flat loaf. To prevent this, use a baguette baking tray or arrange loaves parallel and 7-inches apart on parchment paper lined baking sheet. Push loaves snugly together lifting the paper to form a double-layered wall. Support the long sides with a rolled-up kitchen towel under the parchment. Let rise for 15 minutes.

Preheat oven to 400 degrees F. Bake 15 minutes then brush with egg beaten with 1 teaspoon water to encourage richer browning. Bake an additional 15 minutes or until golden brown.

Cool completely on a wire rack before slicing.

1 cup warm water (105 to 115 degrees F)
1 tablespoon sugar
1 tablespoon active dry yeast

2 tablespoons extra virgin olive oil
1 tablespoon ground flax seed

3 1/3 cups gluten-free flour blend
1/3 cup buckwheat flour, plus more for dusting
2 teaspoons fine sea salt

1 cup gluten-free sourdough starter
2 eggs, beaten

Topping
1 egg, beaten

Salt can inhibit yeast activity. It's important to find the right balance – use enough salt to give rich flavor without compromising the yeast's ability to rise. For best results, use a very active sourdough starter that is making new bubbles with a fresh beer odor. Ground flax seed in this recipe gives a rustic texture and slightly nutty flavor.

Focaccia

prep time	bake time	yield
20 minutes plus 1 hour rise	**30 minutes**	**9-by-13-by-1-inch crust**

Say *Ciao Bella!* to the enchanting fragrant herbs, crispy crust, and tender center of this focaccia. We love this as part of a charcuterie board or in place of garlic bread at any meal. Perfect for sharing with friends — who will never guess it's gluten-free! This recipe doubles easily and is best eaten right away.

Equipment: Stand mixer with dough hook attachment

2 cups gluten-free flour

2/3 cup sorghum flour

1 tablespoon psyllium husk fiber

1 tablespoon sugar

2 teaspoons minced fresh rosemary

1 teaspoon active dry yeast

1/2 teaspoon sea salt

1/2 teaspoon garlic powder

1 cup warm water (105 to 115 degrees F)

1/4 cup extra virgin olive oil

1/4 cup gluten-free sourdough starter

1 tablespoon apple cider vinegar

Toppings

1 teaspoon chopped fresh rosemary, oregano or thyme

1/2 teaspoon flaked sea salt

10 Kalamata olives

5 cherry tomatoes, halved

Arrange a baking mat on 9-by-13-inch rimmed baking sheet or lightly oil baking sheet with olive oil. If using parchment paper, oil the paper.

In a stand mixer bowl with dough hook attachment, whisk flour blend, sorghum flour, psyllium husk, sugar, rosemary, yeast, salt and garlic powder.

To the flour mixture, add warm water, olive oil, starter and apple cider vinegar. Blend on low to combine for 1 minute. Scrape clean the sides and bottom of the bowl with a rubber spatula. Mix on medium for 2 minutes. Dough will be sticky.

Turn out the dough on prepared pan and pat gently into desired shape with oiled fingertips. Leave deep dimples for olive oil to collect.

Cover loosely with plastic wrap and let rise for 60 minutes. Dough will increase in size and bubble up. Make more dimples if desired, drizzle lightly with olive oil and sprinkle generously with fresh herbs, flaky sea salt or other toppings such as black olives and oven dried cherry tomatoes.

Preheat oven to 450 degrees F.

Bake in the top half of the oven 30 minutes or until golden brown. For richer color, finish under a medium broiler for 3 minutes.

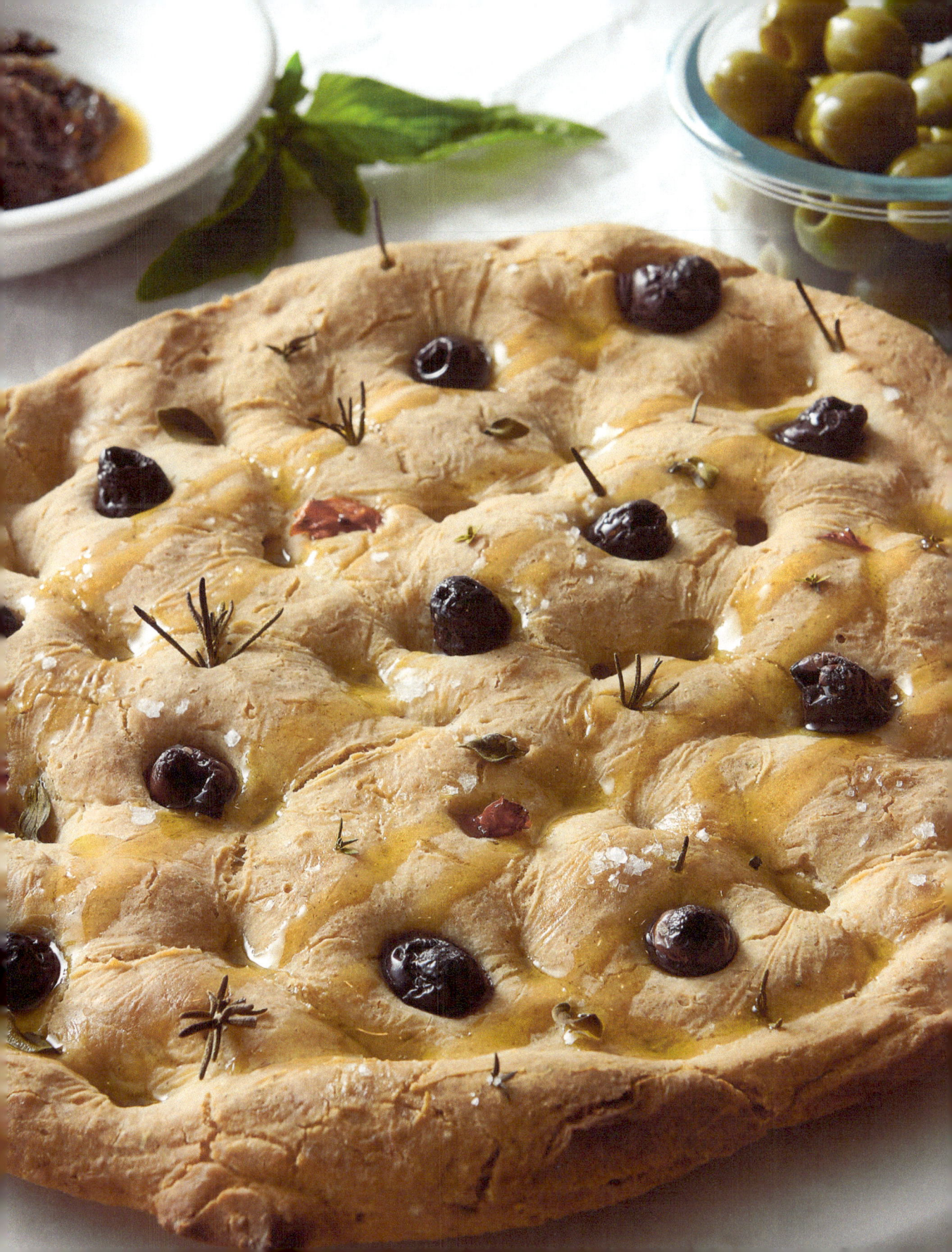

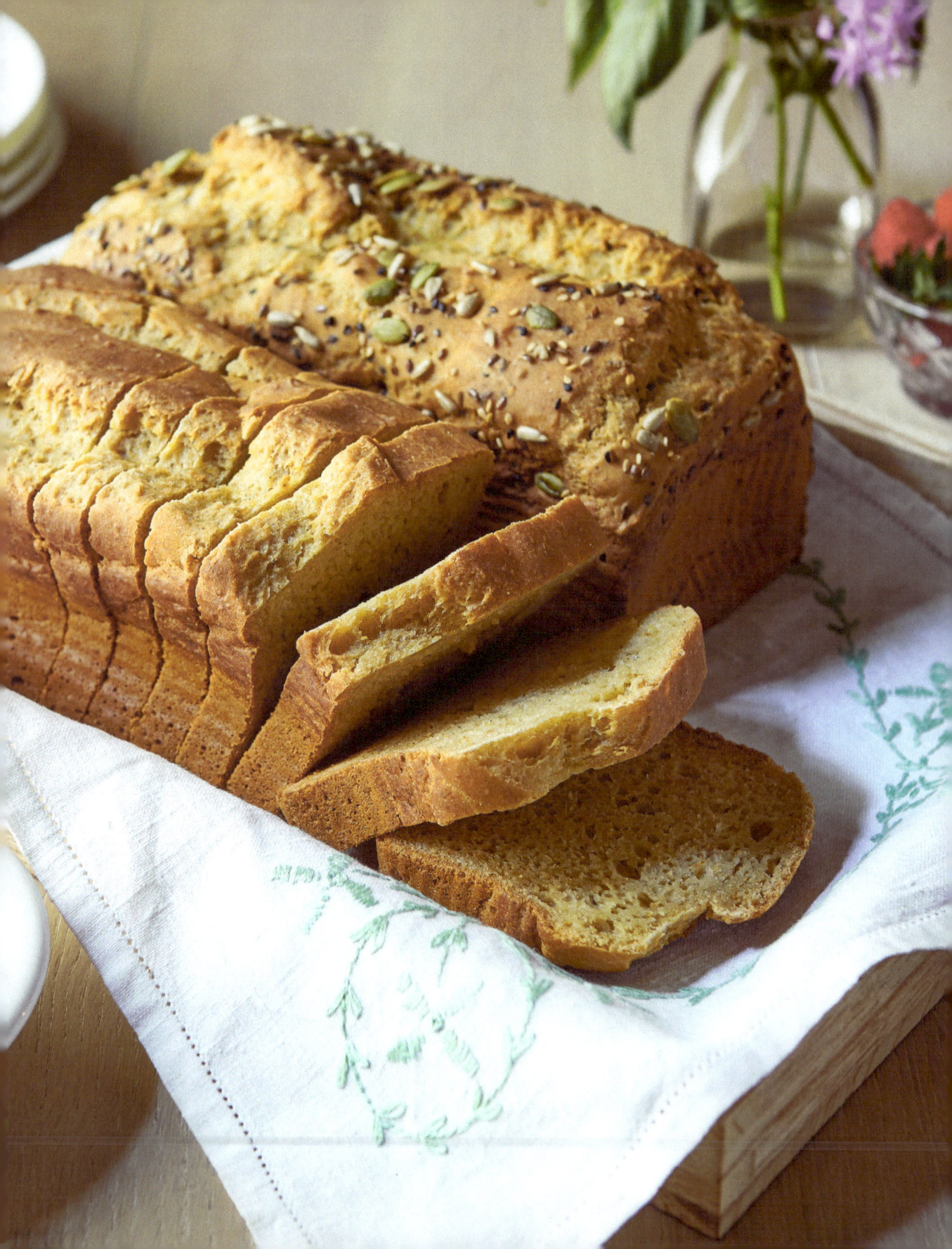

Honey Sandwich Loaf

prep time	bake time	yield
10 minutes plus 1 hour rise	**50 minutes**	**9-by-4-inch Pullman loaf pan**

This bread is the star of the show. No one can tell it is gluten-free! With excellent flavor, sponge and versatility, it's the best recipe for beginners. My husband, a self-professed baking novice, makes this recipe twice a month. It is sure to become a staple recipe in your home.

Equipment: Stand mixer with paddle attachment

Lightly oil pan. In a small glass bowl, dissolve honey in warm water. Stir in yeast and set aside for 10 minutes. A foam should appear on top.

In a medium bowl, whisk the flour blend, ground flax, baking powder, nutritional yeast, psyllium, inulin if using and salt.

In a stand mixer with a paddle attachment, combine eggs, olive oil and apple cider vinegar. Mix on medium speed 20 seconds.

Add starter and honey mixture. Mix on low 20 seconds to combine.

Add the flour mixture. Mix on low for 30 seconds to incorporate. Scrape clean sides and bottom of the bowl with a rubber spatula.

Mix on medium speed for 3 minutes. The batter will be thick and sticky. Stir in fruits and seeds from variations if using, see page 58.

Pour dough mixture into prepared loaf pan. If you desire a smooth crust, gently pat the top smooth with wet fingertips.

Set aside to rise, loosely covered with a clean towel. Rise time will depend on yeast activity and temperature, 30 to 60 minutes. Do not allow the edges of the dough to rise closer than 3/4-inch from the lip of the pan as more rise occurs during baking.

Preheat oven to 375 degrees F with rack arranged in the lower third. Bake 30 minutes. Loosely tent with foil when crust begins to brown. Bake an additional 30 or until internal temperature reaches 210 degrees F.

Cool 20 minutes in pan. Remove and let cool completely on wire rack before slicing. Bread will lose loft and dry out if sliced while warm.

Proof the yeast

1 1/4 cup warm water (105 to 115 degrees F)

1/4 cup honey

1 teaspoon active dry yeast

2 3/4 cup gluten-free flour blend

3 tablespoon ground flax seed

2 tablespoon baking powder

2 tablespoon flaked nutritional yeast

2 tablespoon psyllium husk fiber

1 teaspoon chicory root fiber or inulin (optional)

1 teaspoon salt

2 eggs

1/4 cup extra virgin olive oil, mild tasting (plus more to coat pan)

1 tablespoon apple cider vinegar

1/3 cup gluten-free sourdough starter

Fruit and Seed Loaf

1/2 cup dried cranberries, rehydrated in hot water for 10 minutes, drained

1/2 cup raisins, rehydrated in hot water 10 minutes, drained

2 tablespoons pumpkin seeds

2 tablespoon sunflower seeds

1 tablespoon flax seeds

1 tablespoon sesame seeds

In a small bowl, combine cranberries, raisins, pumpkin seeds, sunflower seeds, flax seeds and sesame seeds.

Reserve 1 tablespoon to sprinkle on top. Stir into batter before pouring into loaf pan.

Vegan option

Replace eggs with 2 tablespoons chia seeds soaked in 1/2 cup warm water. Replace honey with 3 tablespoons of granulated sugar or maple syrup.

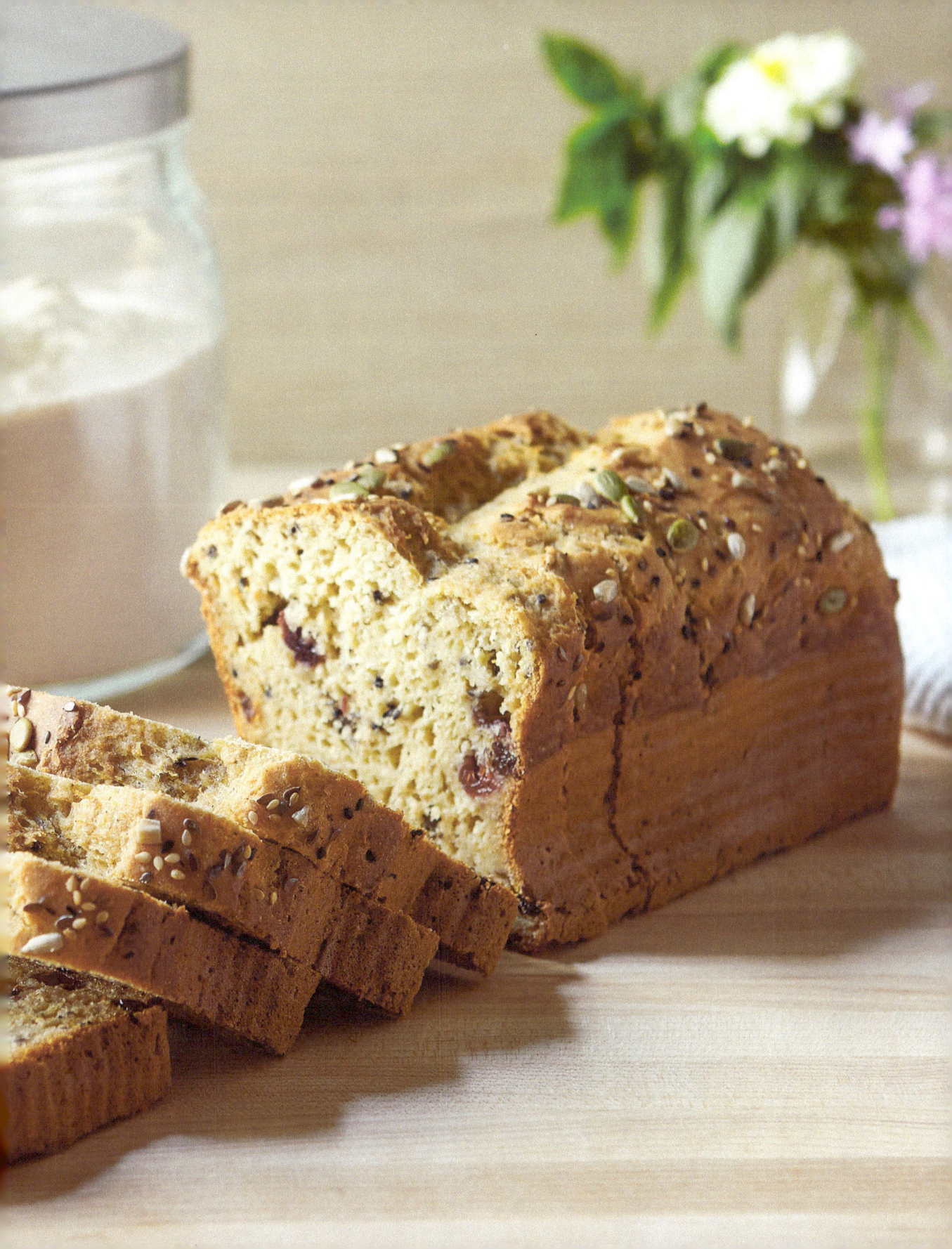

Simple Boule

prep time	bake time	yield
15 minutes plus 12 hours rise	**1 hour 30 minutes**	**9-inch round loaf**

The wait is over! Enjoy the delightfully sour sponge and a chewy crust of this gluten-free boule. For best results, ensure your sourdough starter has been nurtured for at least a month; it should be very active to achieve the appropriate rise. Regularly feeding and using your starter several days leading up to baking will yield the best results. Look for a bubbly, eager starter – this is key to achieving that lovely sponge. Regardless of how the bread rises, you can count on it tasting amazing!

Equipment: Stand mixer with dough hook attachment, Banneton or steep sided bowl, Lidded Dutch oven

1 1/4 cup warm water (105 to 115 degrees F), divided, plus more as needed

3 tablespoons psyllium husk fiber

3 1/4 cup gluten-free flour blend

1 tablespoon sugar (optional)

2 teaspoons fine sea salt

1 teaspoon xanthan gum

3/4 cup gluten-free sourdough starter, visibly active

1 tablespoon extra-virgin olive oil, plus more to coat bowl

1 tablespoon brown rice flour, for dusting

In a small bowl, stir 1 cup warm water with psyllium. Set aside to thicken.

In a stand mixer bowl, whisk flour blend, sugar, salt and xanthan gum. Attach dough hook.

Add thickened psyllium, 1/2 cup warm water, starter and oil. Combine on low to medium 1 minute. A dry dough will form. Scrape clean the sides and bottom of the bowl with rubber spatula.

Mixing on medium, slowly incorporate 1 tablespoon water at a time, up to 1/4 cup, as needed until the flour is combined and dough is smooth, not sticky. The amount of water needed will vary due to humidity, conditions of sourdough starter and moisture content of flour. Mix on medium for 3 minutes. The dough may cling to the sides of the bowl.

Lightly oil a bowl or dust banneton generously with rice flour. With a large rubber spatula, form dough into a ball and transfer to prepared bowl. Cover loosely with lightly oiled plastic wrap and a clean towel allowing room for the dough to rise.

Refrigerate covered bowl overnight or 10 hours. This slow rise allows for rich flavor development.

Handling with care to prevent dough collapse, set dough at room temperature to warm and rise by 40 percent, about 2 hours.

Timing for this bread can be tricky; I usually begin this recipe after lunch to be baked the following morning.

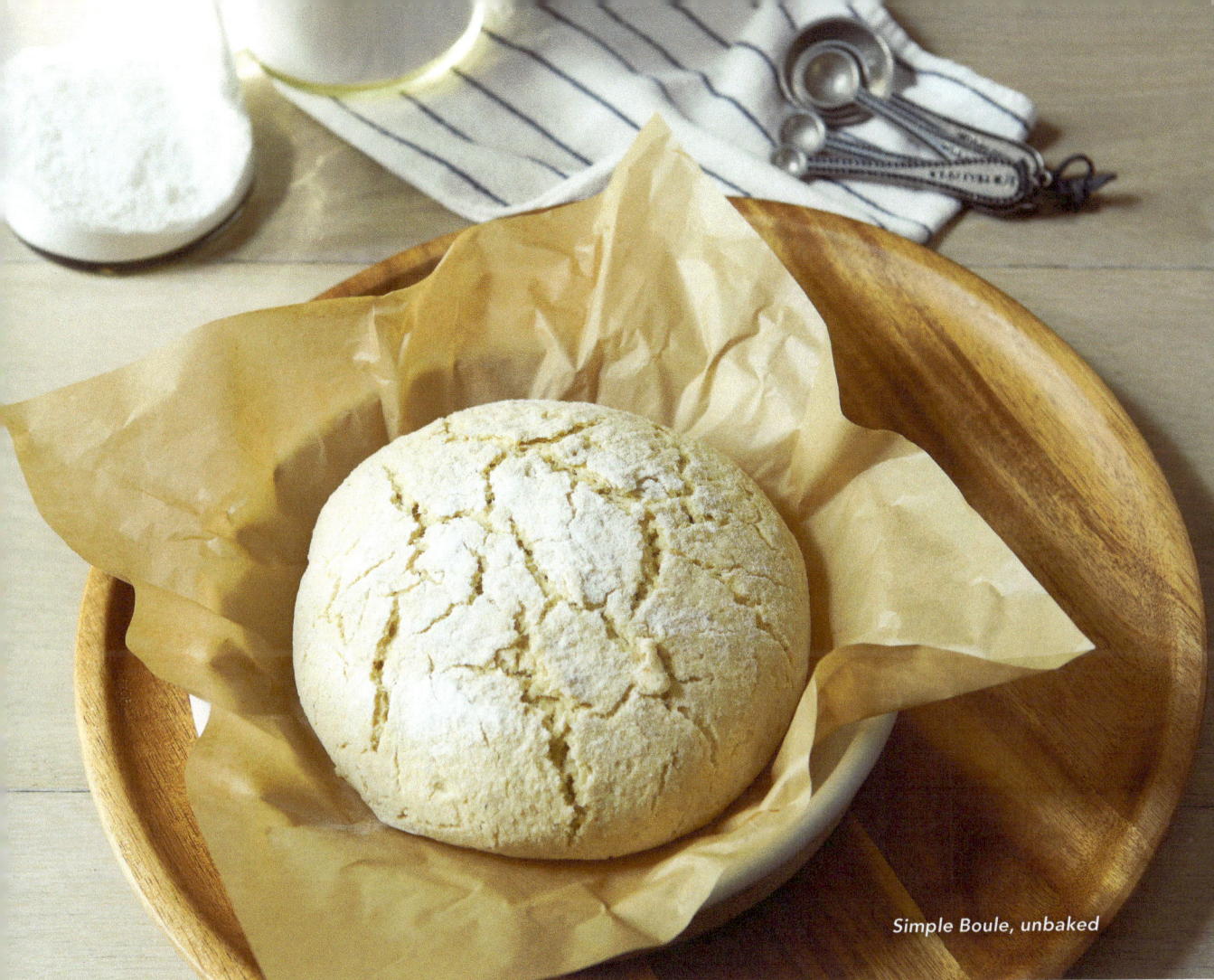

Simple Boule, unbaked

Preheat oven with Dutch oven and lid to 500 degrees F or highest setting with the rack arranged in the lower third.

Score risen dough with 1/2-inch-deep slashes using a sharp knife or bread lame in desired pattern.

Gently place boule and parchment into heated Dutch oven and cover. Bake 60 minutes at 450 degrees F. Remove lid. Poke several deep holes with a metal skewer to allow steam to escape. This prevents gumminess.

Reduce oven to 400 degrees F. Bake an additional 20 to 40 minutes or until internal temperature reaches 210 degrees F. Loosely tent with foil if crust gets dark.

Cool on a wire rack. Bread should cool completely before cutting or it can get gummy. Cut with a serrated bread knife. Store in airtight container at room temperature, this bread does not have a long shelf life at room temperature. Slices and freezes with great results.

Croutons

prep time	bake time
20 minutes	**60 minutes**

Never waste bread again! When making croutons, I prefer to cube leftover bread *before* freezing. These prepared croutons work well for topping a salad, bread pudding or the base for a turkey dressing or stuffing.

Equipment: Sharp bread knife

Leftover gluten-free sourdough bread

Preheat the oven to 250 degrees F with the rack in the lower third of the oven.

Slice bread into 1/2 to 3/4-inch cubes. Arrange in a single layer on a baking sheet. Bake 60 minutes, tossing occasionally, until thoroughly dry.

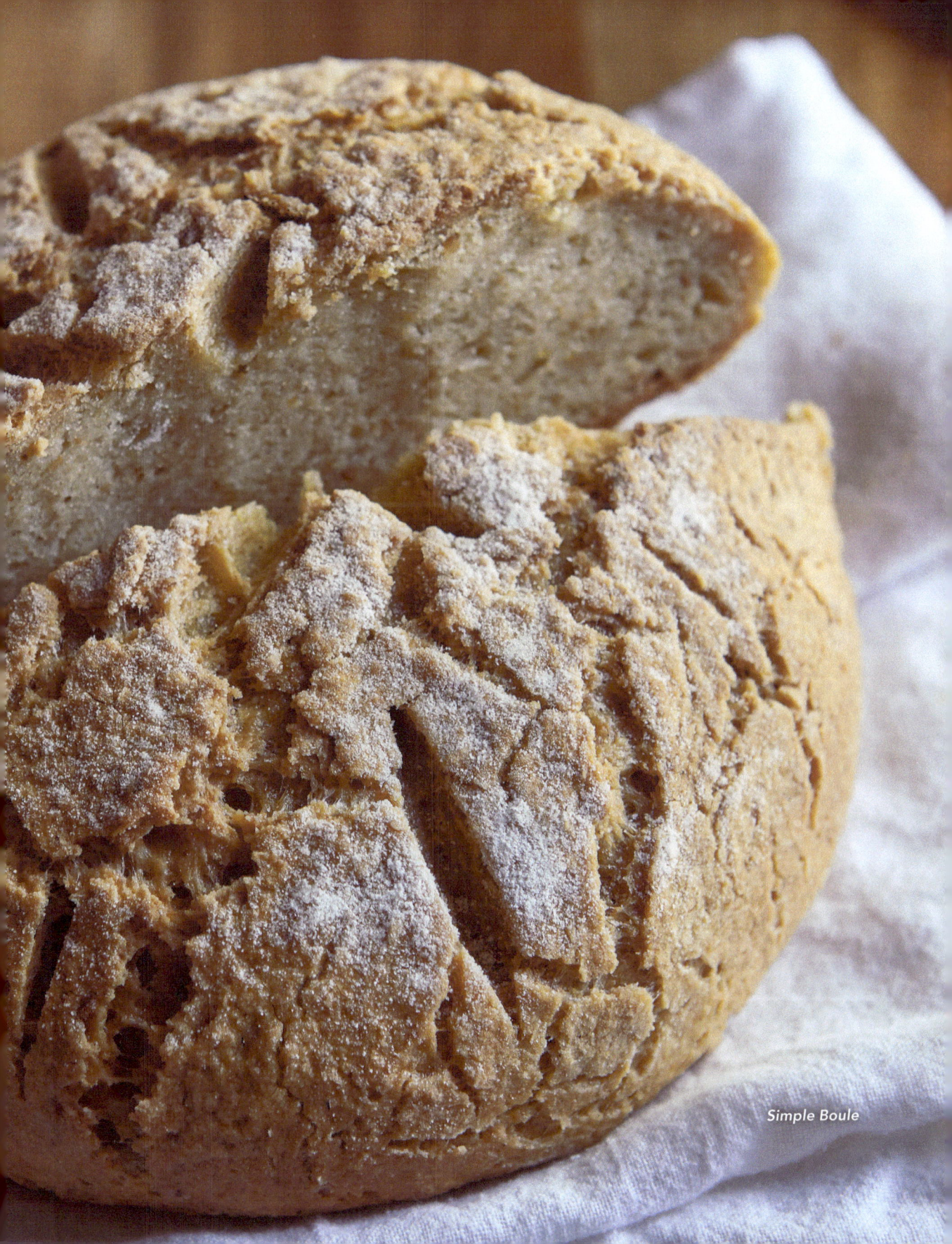

Simple Boule

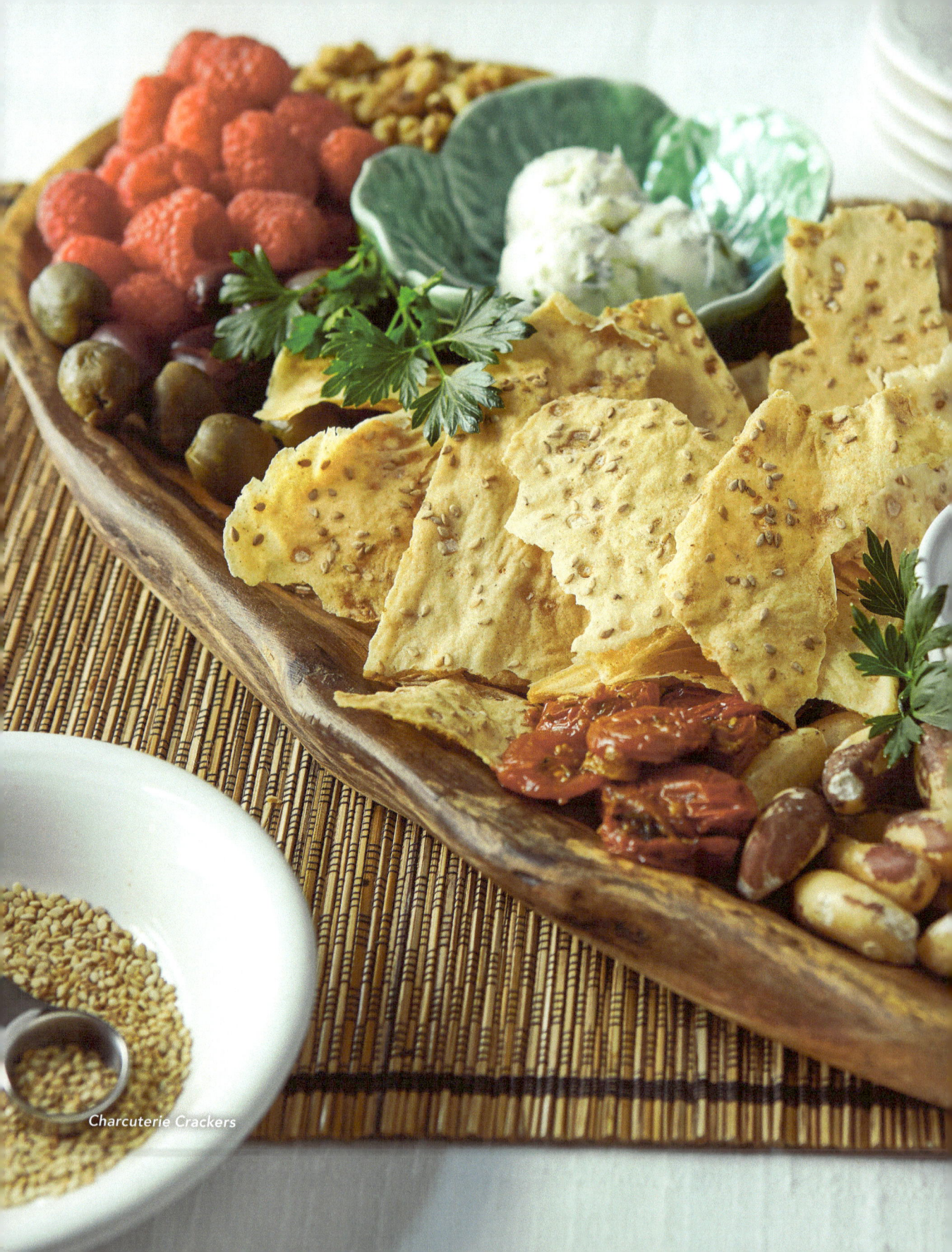

Charcuterie Crackers

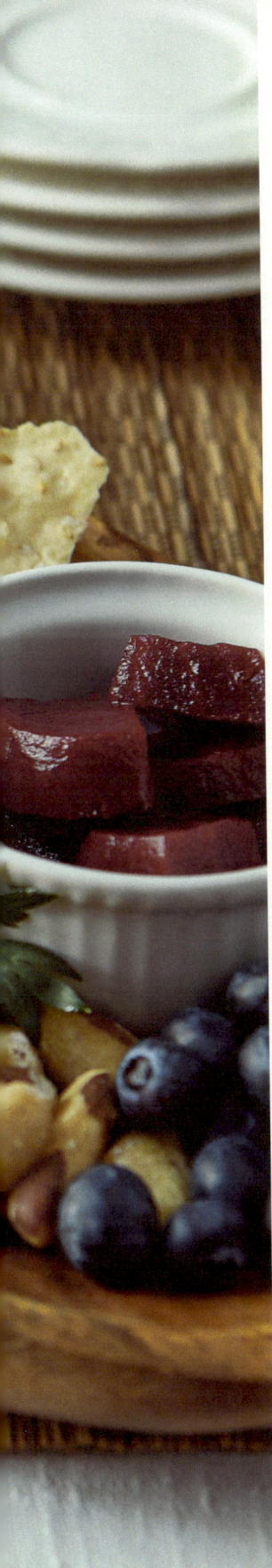

Snacks

I can't help but feeling a little wasteful throwing out sourdough discard, which is why I love making these snack recipes again and again. From sweet and satisfying Cinnamon Sugar Crackers to savory Popovers, this chapter offers the perfect treats to curb your snack cravings or impress your guests. These homemade snacks are also a great way to replace store-bought processed foods and take control of what you're eating. Baking with sourdough discard adds a unique depth of flavor and nutrients that store-bought options can't match. When you make your own snacks, you know exactly what goes into them, ensuring healthier choices for you and your family. I really hope you enjoy these snacks as much as I loved creating them!

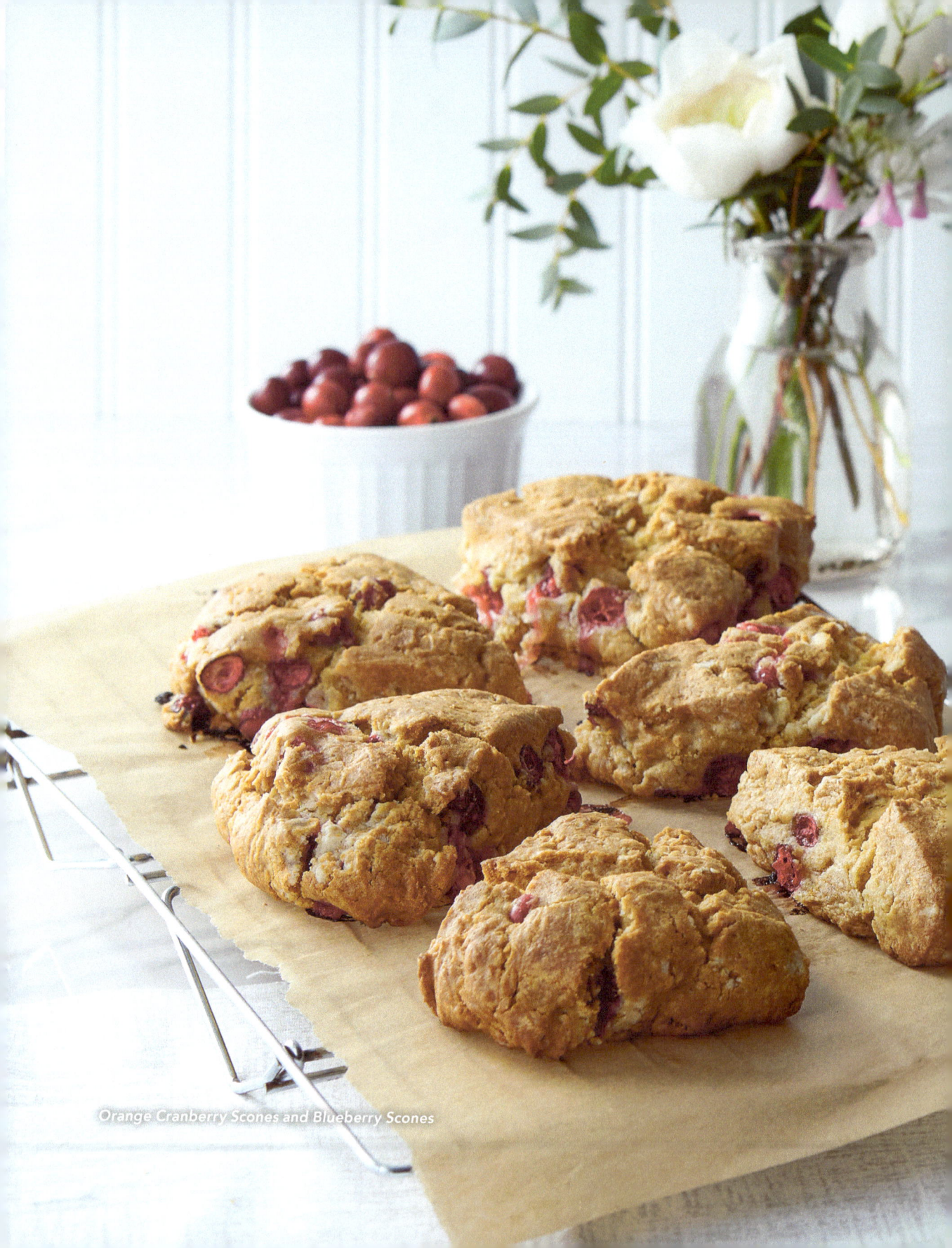

Orange Cranberry Scones and Blueberry Scones

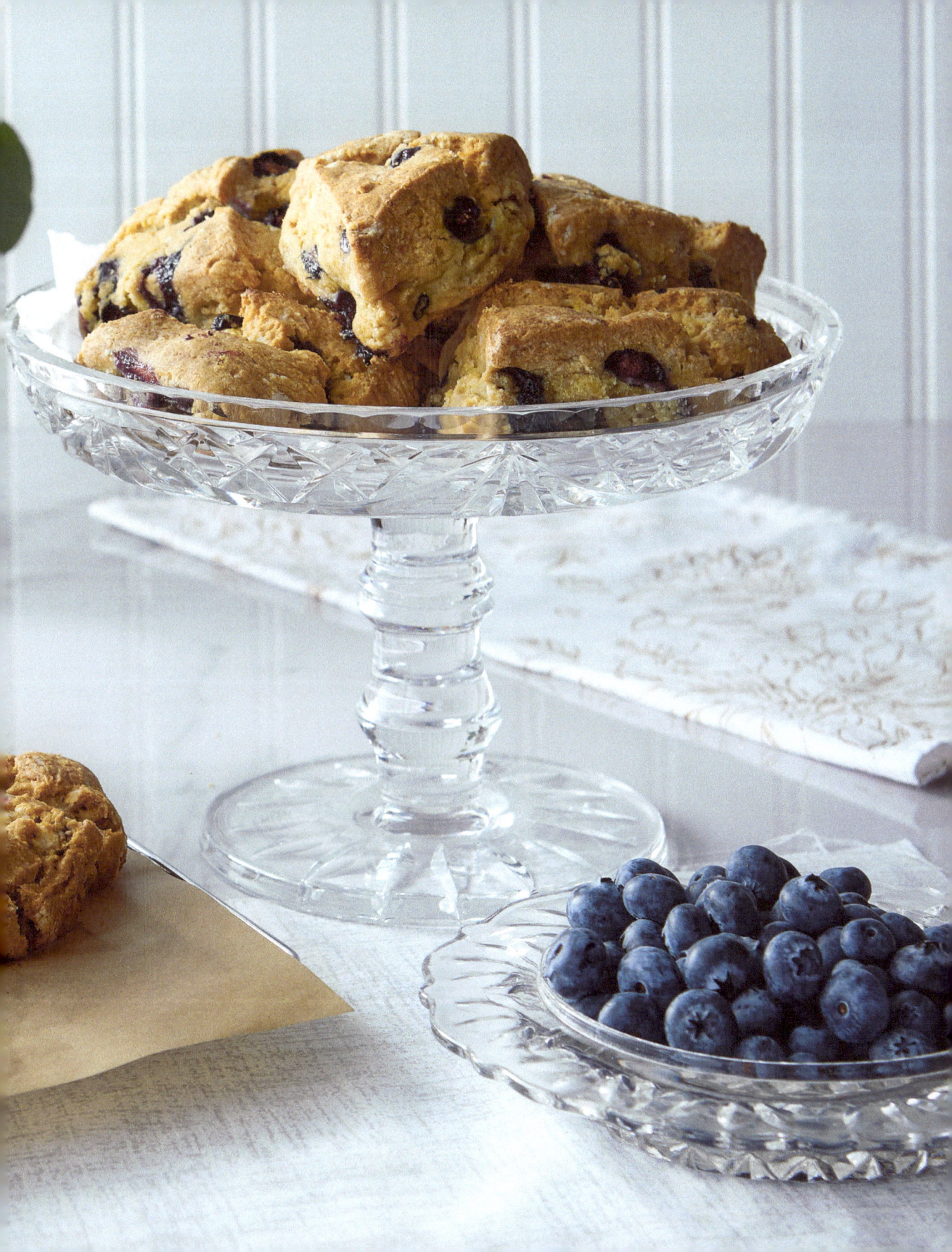

Blueberry Scones

prep time	bake time	yield
10 minutes plus	**40 minutes**	**6 large or 8 small scones**
30 minutes chill		

For over thirty years, I've had a hobby of sampling any variations of scone I could find, but one gluten-free high-tea experience in London truly inspired me. Their adorable, bite-sized gluten-free fruit scones were a delight. I keep several scones frozen for a not-too-sweet and fluffy treat that's ready to bake-up anytime. These freeze brilliantly after baking as well!

Equipment: Food processor with dough blade, Bench scraper

1 cup gluten-free flour blend, plus more for dusting

1/2 cup almond flour

1/2 cup tapioca starch

2 tablespoons sugar

1 tablespoon baking powder

1 teaspoon lightly packed lemon zest

1/2 teaspoon baking soda

1/2 teaspoon salt

1/2 cup milk alternative

1/4 cup gluten-free sourdough starter

1/2 cup (1 stick) vegan butter, diced and frozen

3/4 cup frozen blueberries

In a small bowl, combine milk and starter. Set aside.

In food processor with dough blade, pulse flour blend, almond flour, tapioca starch, sugar, baking powder, lemon zest, baking soda and salt to combine.

Add frozen butter and pulse to make a crumble (see image p. 97-98). Stop frequently to stir excess flour from corners. Transfer to medium mixing bowl.

Stir milk mixture into flour crumble to form a loose ball. Gently fold in blueberries. Working quickly, turn onto flour dusted surface. Use a bench scraper to shape dough into a 2 1/2-inch tall circle. Wrap with plastic wrap and freeze 30 minutes.

Cut into 6 or 8 triangles using a single downward slice, a sawing motion will inhibit the rise. Separate slices 1-inch apart. Cover and freeze for at least 6 hours or up to 1 month in airtight container. Freezing the dough maintains loft and shape when baking.

Preheat oven to 400 degrees F. Arrange frozen scones 1-inch apart on a rimmed baking sheet lined with baking mat or parchment paper. Bake 40 minutes or until light golden brown. Serve warm.

Orange Cranberry Scones

Substitute milk alternative for 1/4 cup milk alternative mixed with 1/4 cup orange juice (about the juice of 1 medium orange). Substitute blueberries with 1 cup fresh cranberries or 1/2 cup dried cranberries. Substitute lemon zest with zest of 1 medium orange. If using fresh cranberries, increase sugar to 1/4 cup to balance tartness.

Follow instructions for blueberry scones.

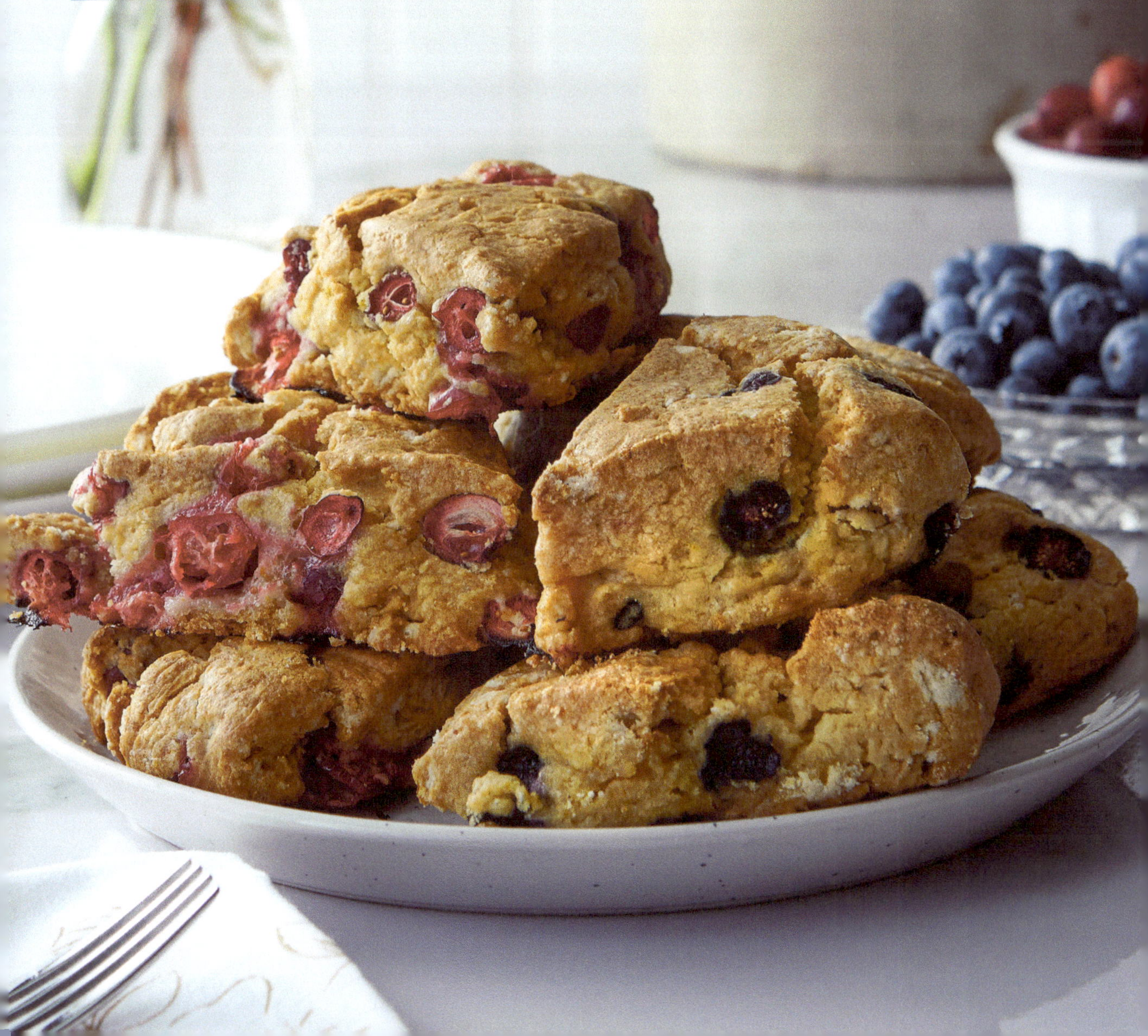

Cinnamon Sugar Crackers

prep time	bake time	yield
10 minutes plus	**20 minutes**	**4 dozen 1 1/2-inch crackers**
20 minutes chill		

These crackers are a heartwarming reminder of a certain popular and beloved breakfast cereal. Enjoy them alone as a wholesome snack or elevate your next charcuterie board. Their sturdy texture is perfect for dipping. This recipe is a great way for beginners to get comfortable with a no-fail dough.

Equipment: Rolling pin

Topping
1 tablespoon sugar
1 teaspoon Ceylon cinnamon

Crackers
1/4 cup gluten-free flour blend
1/4 cup sorghum flour
1 tablespoon sugar
1 teaspoon Ceylon cinnamon

1/2 cup gluten-free sourdough starter
3 tablespoons vegan butter, melted

Topping
In a small bowl, whisk the sugar and cinnamon. Set aside.

Crackers
In a medium bowl, whisk flour blend, sorghum flour, sugar and cinnamon. Add sourdough starter and butter. Stir to form a smooth ball. Wrap the ball tightly with plastic wrap or Bee's Wrap and refrigerate for 20 minutes. Dough may be refrigerated for up to 24 hours.
Preheat oven to 375 degrees F.
On a baking mat or parchment cut to fit a 9-by-13-inch baking sheet, cover dough with plastic wrap. Roll evenly to 1/8-inch thick. Cut into 1 1/2-inch squares using a rolling pizza cutter. Poke each square with a fork to prevent bubbling up. Sprinkle with topping. Transfer to baking sheet.
Bake 15 minutes. Rotate baking sheet and bake an additional 10 to 15 minutes or until lightly golden. Crackers will continue to darken while cooling. Sprinkle with more cinnamon and sugar, if desired. Cool 10 minutes then break the crackers apart. Store in airtight container.

Serve cinnamon sugar crackers with sweet cream cheese dip.
Refrigerate dip in airtight container for up to 3 months.

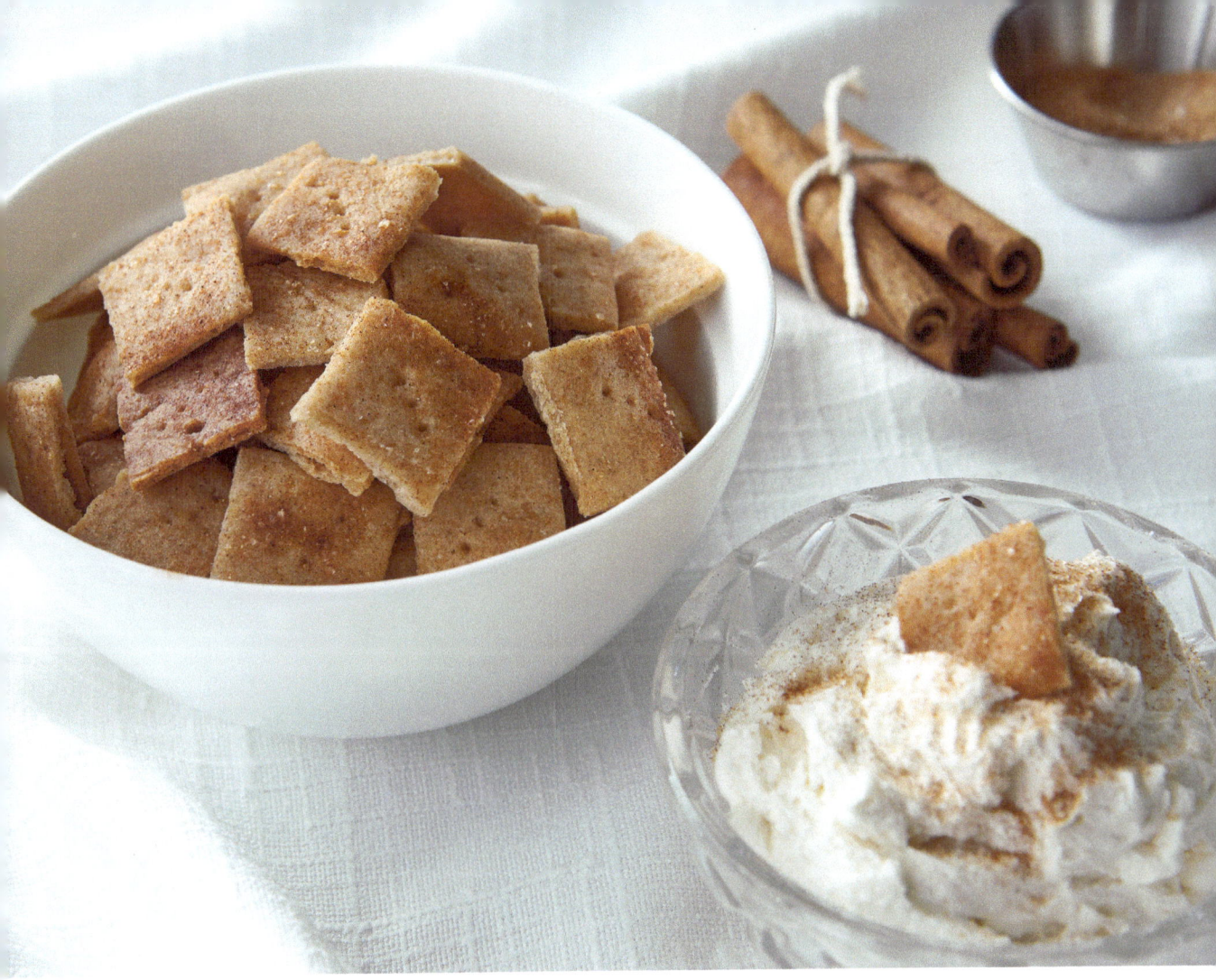

Sweet Cream Cheese Dip

Equipment: Stand mixer with whisk attachment

In a stand mixer with whisk attachment, blend butter and 1 cup powdered sugar on low. Add milk, lemon juice, vinegar, salt, and another cup of powdered sugar.

Mix on low to prevent powdered sugar from dusting up then increase to medium. Add more powdered sugar to sweeten and thicken or add more milk to thin, until dip is sweet, smooth and fluffy.

1/2 cup (1 stick) vegan butter

3 cups powdered sugar, sifted

2 tablespoons milk alternative

2 teaspoons fresh lemon juice

2 teaspoons apple cider vinegar

1/4 teaspoon sea salt

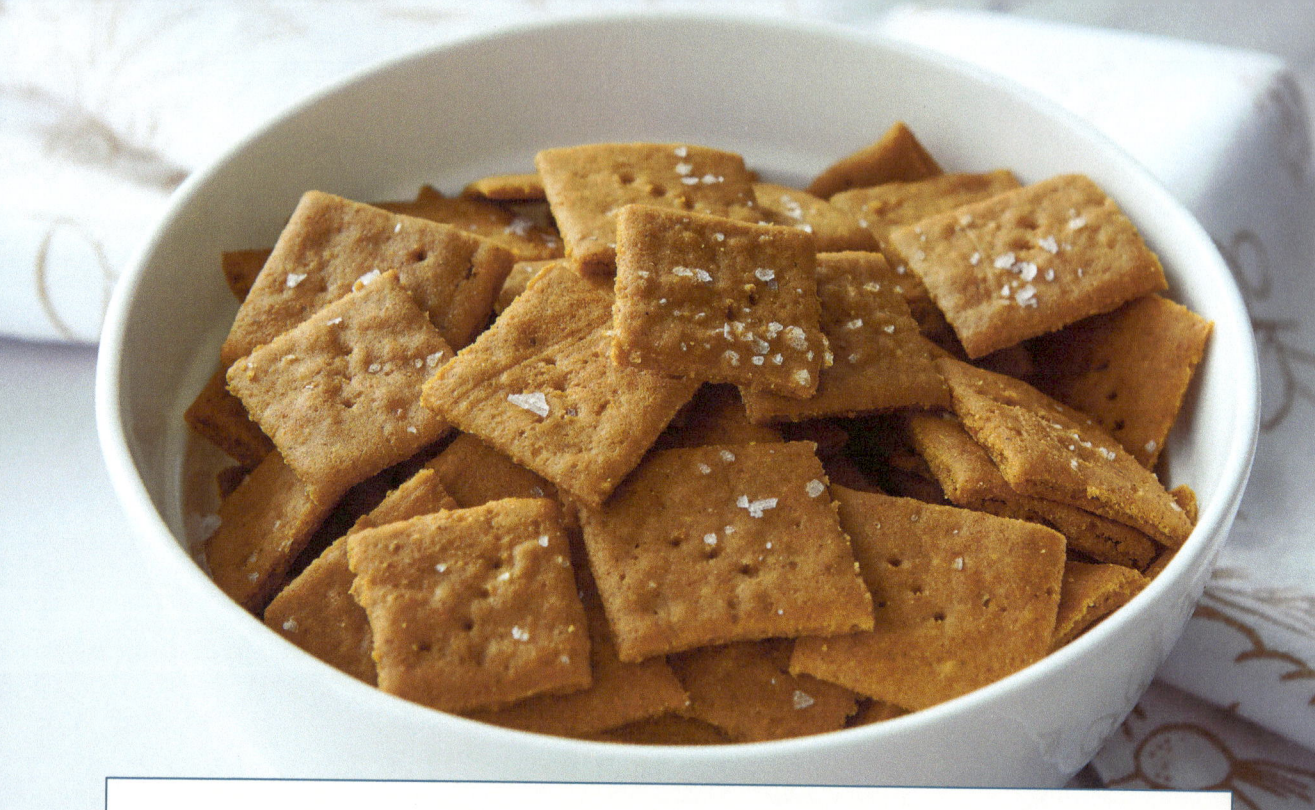

Cheddar Crackers

Variation of the Cinnamon Sugar Crackers

1/4 cup gluten-free flour blend

1/4 cup sorghum flour

2 tablespoons nutritional yeast

1/2 teaspoon baking soda

1/2 teaspoon paprika

1/2 teaspoon salt

1/2 teaspoon turmeric

1/2 cup gluten-free sourdough starter

3 tablespoons vegan butter, melted and room temperature

Topping

1 teaspoon flaked sea salt

Follow instructions for Cinnamon Sugar Crackers. Sprinkle with flaked sea salt before baking. Be careful not to overbake as crackers will continue to darken while cooling.

Charcuterie Crackers

prep time	bake time	yield
5 minutes	**30 minutes to 1 hour**	**About 2 cups**

Hands-down, this is the easiest way to use discard! You could say this cracker is like a leavened, gluten-free, non-Kosher cousin of matzah (matzo) crackers. They are no-fuss, oddly addictive crackers with a crispy texture with mildly tangy flavor. Want a thicker cracker? Simply spread the starter thicker and increase baking time.

Preheat oven to 350 degrees F. Line 13-by-9-inch baking sheet with parchment paper or baking mat.

Pour the starter on parchment paper and spread thin and evenly to about 1/8-inch thick or to desired thickness. Thickness and hydration of the starter directly affects baking time.

Sprinkle with salt and toppings as desired.

Bake 30 minutes or until completely dry and light golden brown.

If edges dry and darken before the center, break off dry areas and return to oven.

1 cup gluten-free sourdough starter

Flake sea salt

Variations

1 teaspoon sesame seeds

1/2 teaspoon flavored flake sea salt

1/2 teaspoon minced fresh rosemary

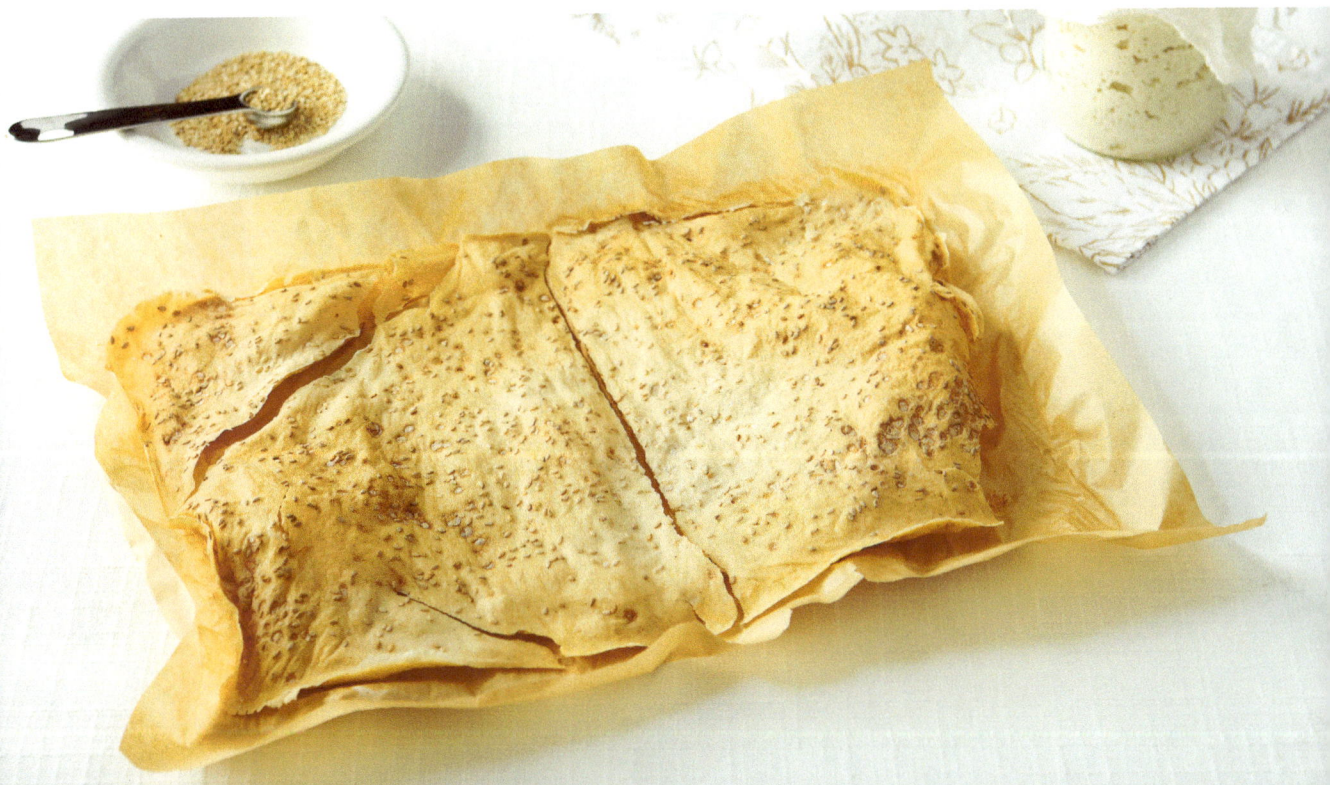

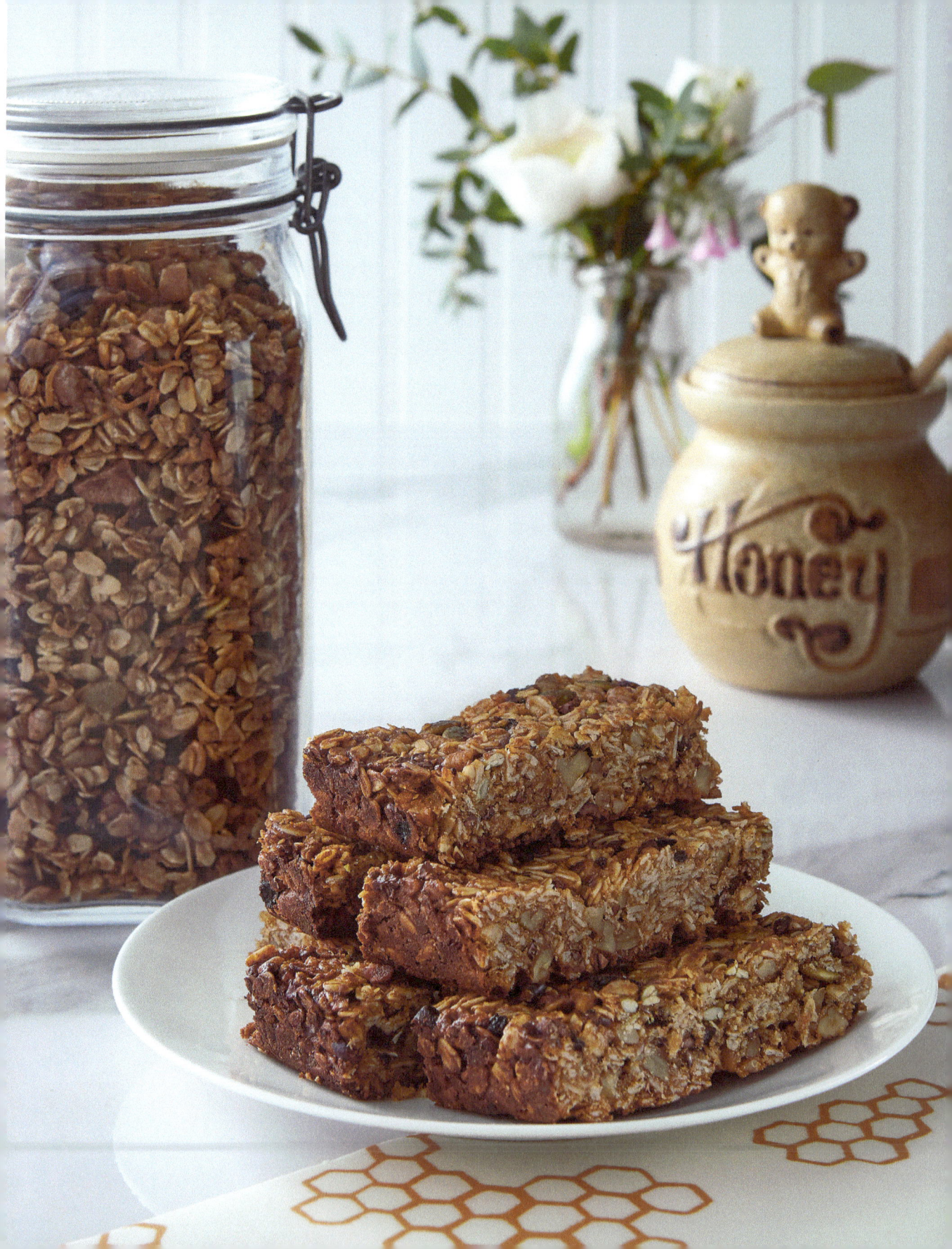

Granola

prep time	bake time	yield
10 minutes	**40 minutes**	**8 cups**

Say goodbye to store-bought granola! My husband loves this granola as a cereal with oat milk and fresh fruit, while I prefer it as a topping for vegan Greek yogurt. This recipe is fully customizable – feel free to add or swap ingredients to suit your taste. You can also easily transform it into granola bars!

Preheat oven to 350 degrees F. Prepare a large (15-inch-by-21-inch) rimmed baking sheet with baking mat or parchment paper.

In a large bowl, combine oats, nuts, coconut, pumpkin seeds, hemp seeds, flax seeds, cinnamon and salt. Add oil, honey and starter. Stir to mix well. Spread in an even layer filling the baking sheet.

Bake 20 minutes. Stir and bake an additional 20 minutes or until all the granola is deep golden brown.

Stir in dry fruit if using, while granola is warm. Cool completely before serving.

3 cups gluten-free rolled oats

2 cups chopped nuts, pecans, walnuts, pistachios, almonds or peanuts

1/2 cup unsweetened coconut flakes

1/4 cup pumpkin seeds

2 tablespoons hemp seeds (optional)

1 tablespoon flax seeds

1 teaspoon Ceylon cinnamon

1 teaspoon sea salt

1/2 cup avocado oil

1/2 cup honey or maple syrup

1/2 cup gluten-free sourdough starter

1/2 to 1 cup raisins, dried cranberries, currants or dates, chopped (optional)

Granola Bars

To above recipe: Decrease oil to 1/4 cup. Add 1/2 cup peanut or almond butter, 1/2 cup mini dairy-free chocolate chips or cacao nibs and 1 teaspoon vanilla.

Line 9-by-13-by-3-inch cake pan with parchment paper. Press mixture firmly using large rubber spatula, oiled hands or piece of parchment paper.

Bake at 350 degrees F for 40 minutes or until golden brown. Cool completely before cutting into bars. Store in airtight container.

Pancakes

prep time	bake time	yield
45 minutes	**8 minutes per pancake**	**10 4-inch pancakes**

Gluten-free can taste great – especially on Pancake Day! These pancakes are thick and fluffy, reminiscent of the enormous flapjacks from the 1970s children's book *Cloudy with a Chance of Meatballs*. While I've never flipped one onto my son's head – yet, they are sure to be a huge hit on your breakfast table!

1 cup gluten-free flour blend

1 teaspoon baking powder

1 cup gluten-free sourdough starter

1 cup stirred full-fat, unsweetened coconut milk

2 eggs, beaten

2 tablespoons maple syrup

1 tablespoon extra-virgin olive oil or avocado oil

1/2 teaspoon vanilla

1/4 teaspoon salt

In a medium bowl, whisk flour blend and baking powder. Add starter and coconut milk and combine with a Danish dough hook or rubber spatula. The mixture will be thick.

In a small bowl, combine eggs, maple syrup, oil, vanilla and salt. Stir into the flour mixture. Cover loosely with a kitchen towel to sit at room temperature for 30 minutes until fluffy and bubbly.

Heat griddle or cast-iron skillet on medium-high heat. Pour 1/4 cup batter on a hot lightly oiled griddle. The pancakes will form a light and tangy crispy crust if the skillet is hot enough. Flip when bubbles have surfaced and popped, about 4 minutes. Cook second side for 4 minutes or until golden brown. For best results, flip once and never press down on the pancake.

Store in airtight freezer bag or container with pieces of parchment paper between pancakes. Freeze leftover coconut milk in an ice cube tray. Substitute coconut milk with any milk for delicious pancakes, but they may be less fluffy.

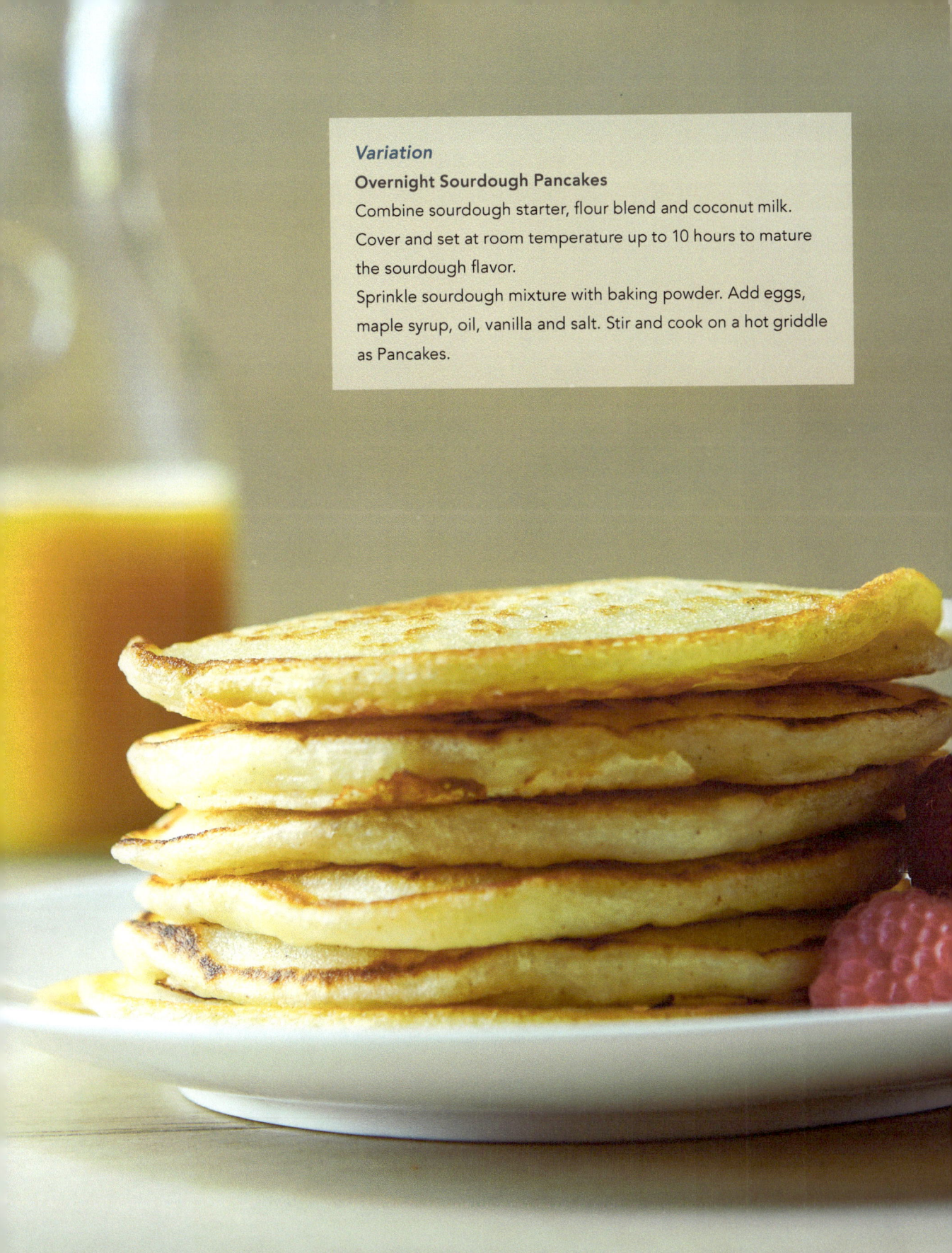

Variation

Overnight Sourdough Pancakes

Combine sourdough starter, flour blend and coconut milk.
Cover and set at room temperature up to 10 hours to mature
the sourdough flavor.

Sprinkle sourdough mixture with baking powder. Add eggs,
maple syrup, oil, vanilla and salt. Stir and cook on a hot griddle
as Pancakes.

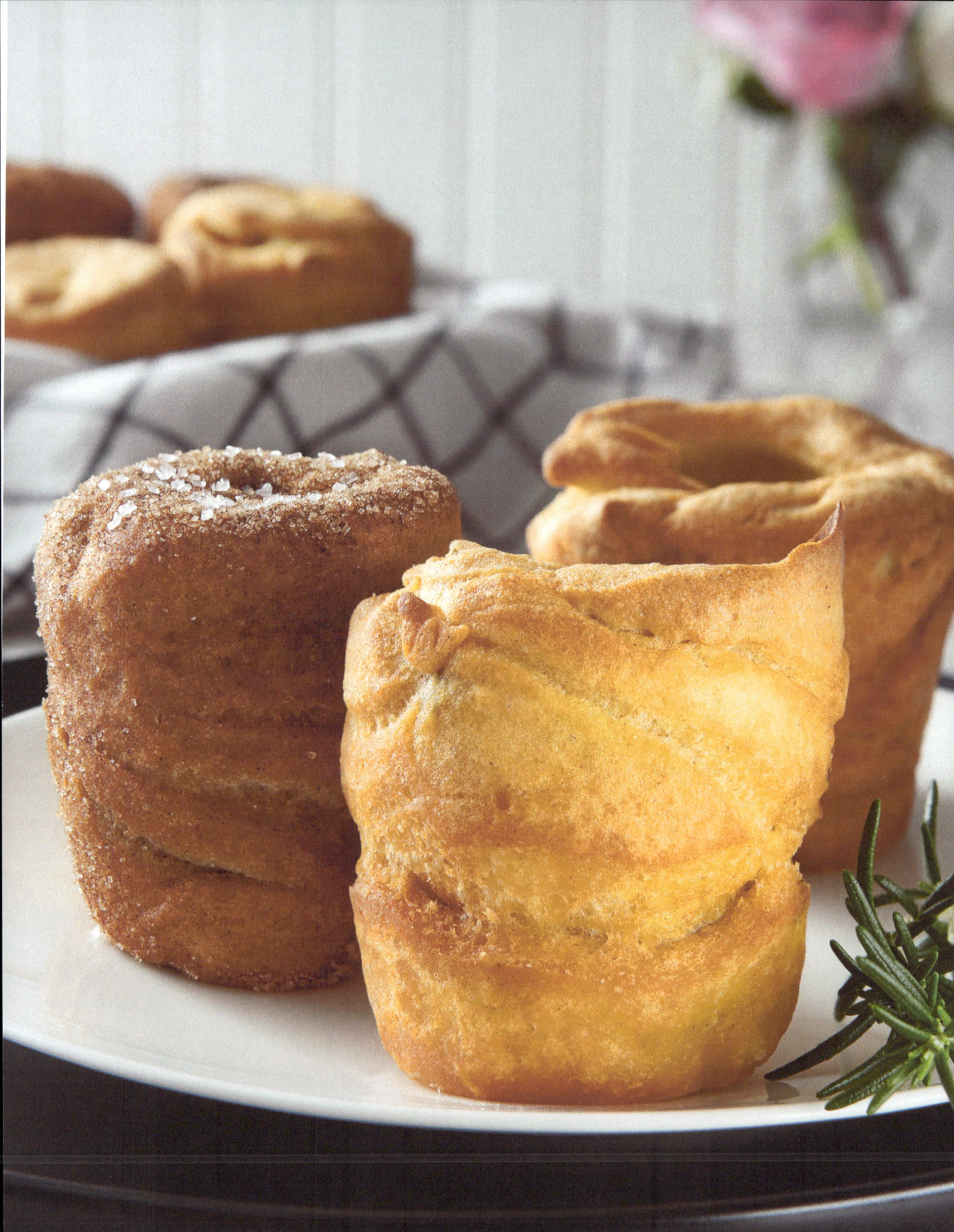

Popovers

prep time	bake time	yield
25 minutes	**30 minutes**	**4 popovers**

I find popovers to be steeped in mystery and prestige, evoking images of elegant dinners and black bow ties. These puffed-up treats, with their crispy exterior and airy interior, feel sophisticated but are surprisingly easy to make! Perfect for brunch, a snack or an elevated side when entertaining, these popovers will impress guests and leave them asking for the recipe! Double this recipe with ease.

Equipment: Popover pan (3-inch cupcake pan with steeply angled sides)

In medium bowl with a pouring spout, whisk flour blend and salt. Whisk in eggs, starter and milk until smooth. Refrigerate 20 minutes. Preheat oven to 450 degrees F.

To 4 popover cups add 1 tablespoon butter each. Set in oven until bubbling hot. Carefully fill cups 3/4 full of batter.

Bake 20 minutes. Decrease oven to 350 degrees F. Bake additional 10 to 20 minutes or until golden brown. Serve hot.

1 cup gluten-free flour blend
1/2 teaspoon fine sea salt

2 eggs, beaten
1/2 cup gluten-free sourdough starter
1/2 cup milk alternative

4 tablespoons vegan butter

Variations

Sweet Cinnamon Popover
Add 3 teaspoons sugar and 1 teaspoon cinnamon to batter. For a churro-like popover, brush warm popovers with melted butter and toss in a cinnamon and sugar mixture.

Savory Popover
Add 2 teaspoons minced fresh rosemary to batter.

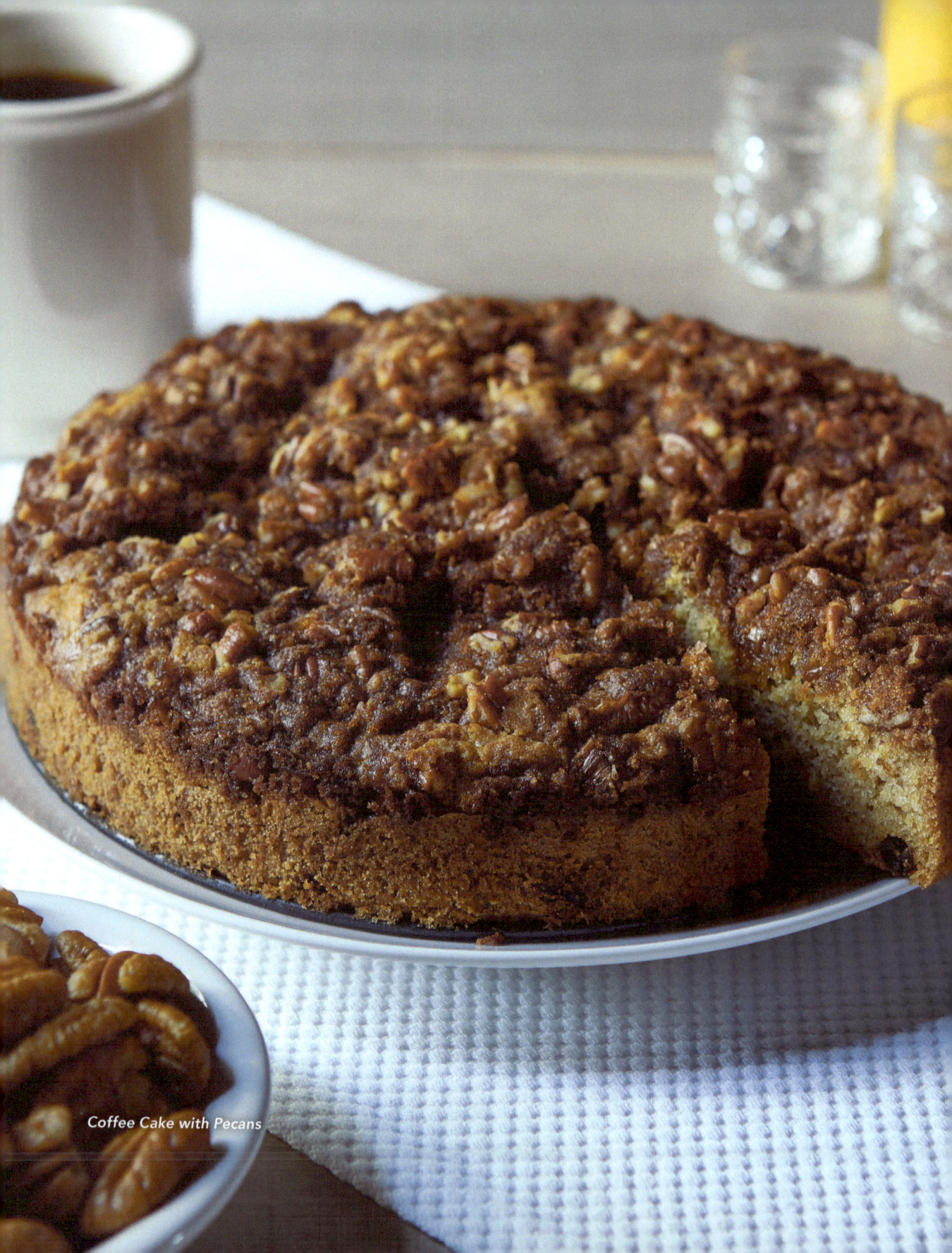

Coffee Cake with Pecans

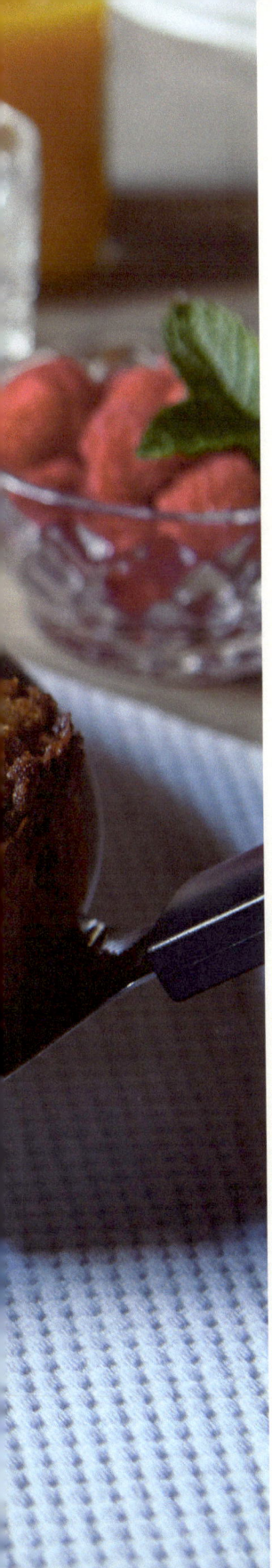

Sweets

Sourdough starter isn't just for savory breads – it adds delicate depth of flavor and moisture to gluten-free desserts, too. In this chapter, you'll discover how sourdough can elevate classic sweets like Blackberry Cobbler, Blueberry Muffins, rich Chocolate Bundt Cake, Coffee Cake with Pecans, delicate Crepes and zesty Lemon Pound Cake. Baking with sourdough starter not only enhances flavor but also adds nutrition and creates a tender crumb. While we don't indulge in sweets every day, these treats offer a more wholesome way to satisfy your sweet tooth. I can't decide if I prefer the Chocolate Bundt Cake or the Crepes more. Grab your sourdough starter and find out which dessert becomes your new favorite!

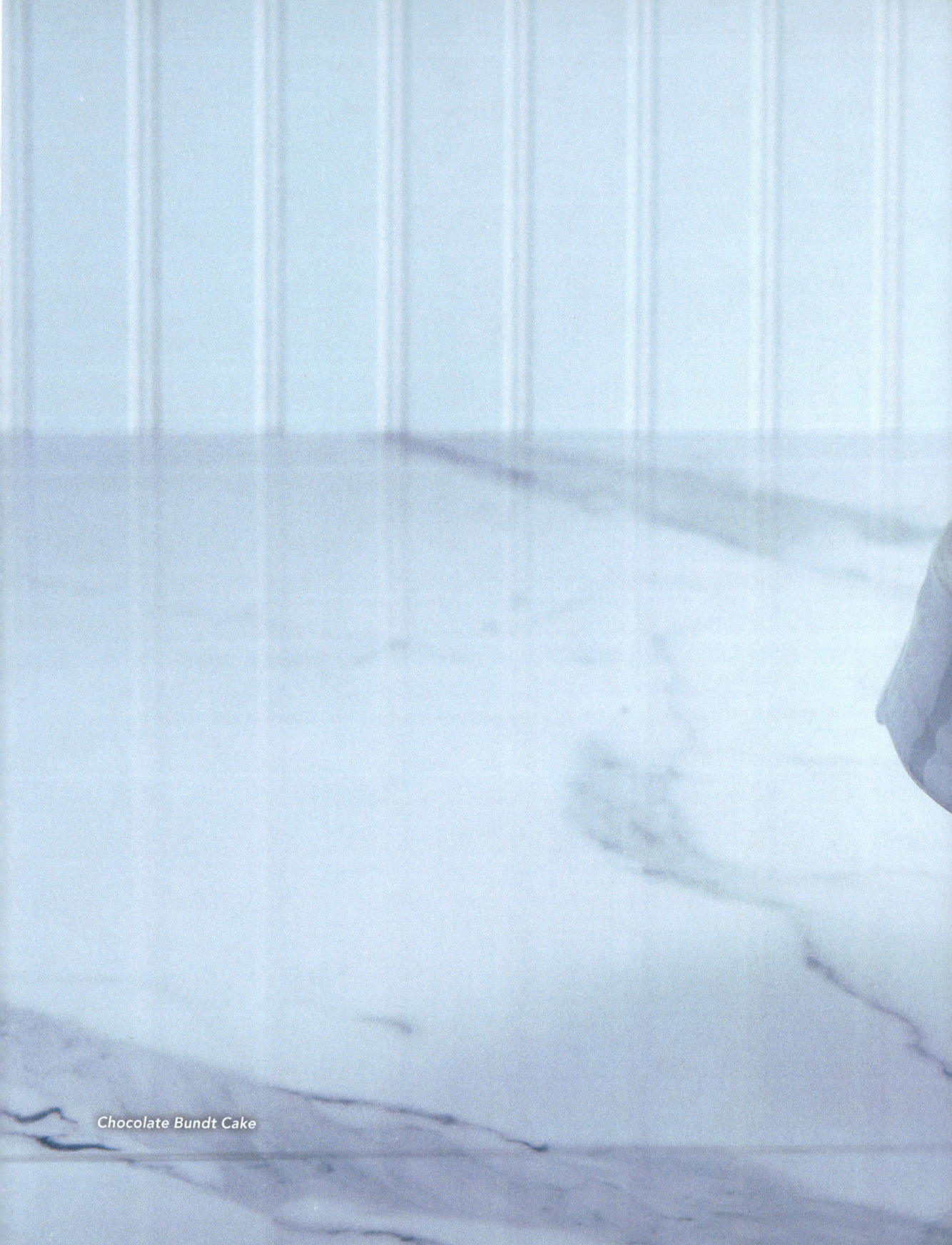

Chocolate Bundt Cake

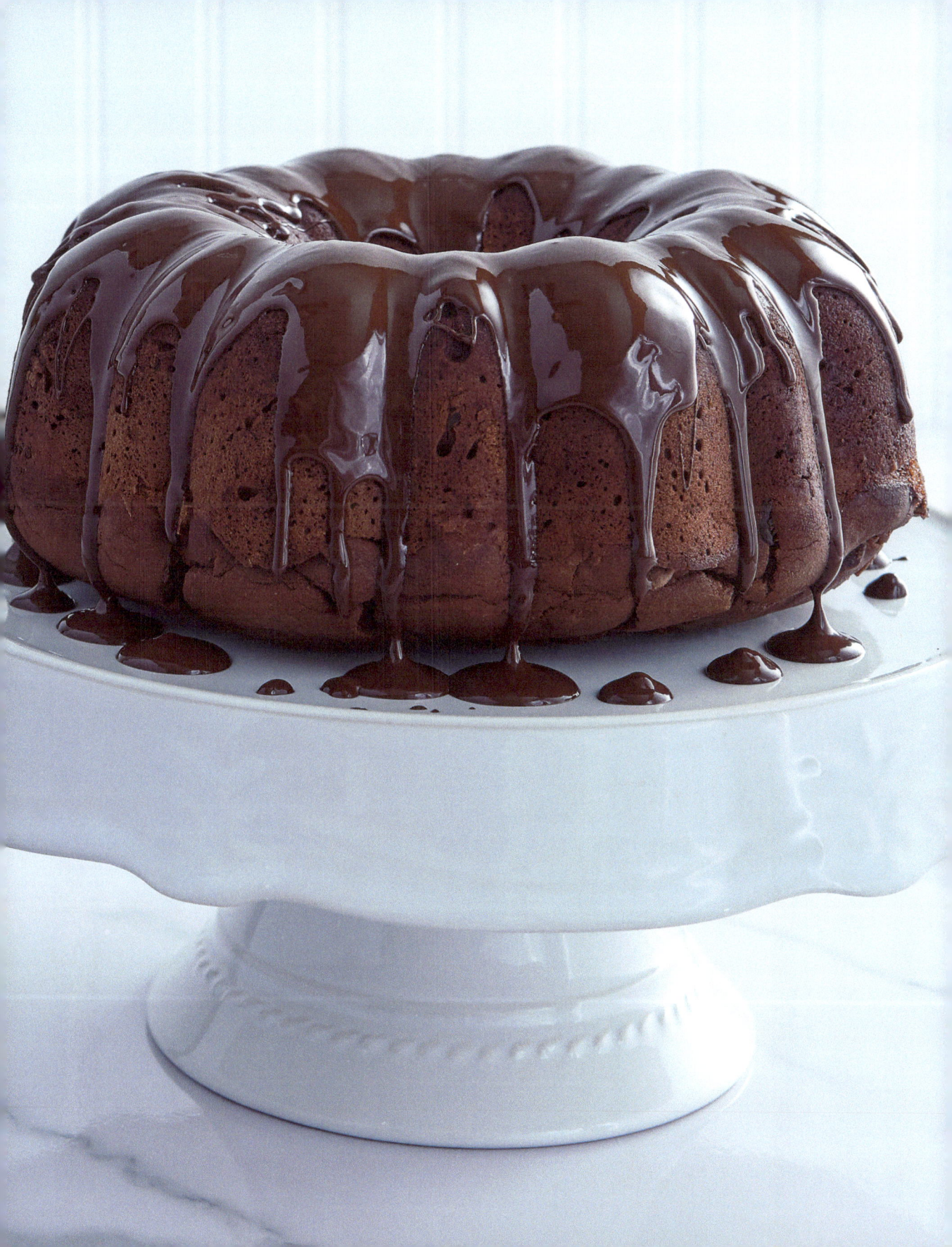

Blackberry Cobbler

prep time	bake time	yield
15 minutes	**60 minutes**	**8-by-8-inch glass dish**

Nothing says summer in Texas quite like a sweet and comforting cobbler. This recipe has been loved by my family for years, especially at our gatherings. Inspired by a version I created in 2006, this is a favorite my mother-in-law frequently requests – and for good reason! The combination of sweet fruit and buttery topping makes it a crowd-pleaser every time.

3 cups (12 ounces) fresh blackberries

1/4 cup sugar

1 teaspoon arrowroot powder

1/2 cup milk alternative, unsweetened

2 teaspoons apple cider vinegar

3 tablespoons vegan butter, melted

1/2 cup gluten-free flour blend

1/2 cup sorghum flour or millet flour

2 teaspoons baking powder

1/2 teaspoon salt

1/4 cup gluten-free sourdough starter

In a medium bowl, combine blackberries, sugar and arrowroot. Set aside.

In a small glass, stir milk and vinegar. Set aside.

Preheat the oven to 400 degrees F. Melt butter in 8-by-8-inch glass baking dish.

In a medium bowl, whisk flour blend, sorghum flour, baking powder and salt. Add milk mixture, starter and hot melted butter to flour mixture. Whisk to combine. The batter will be slightly bubbly and smell like fresh homemade biscuits. Spread blackberries and any syrup that developed in the baking dish. Spoon batter over blackberries to cover.

Bake 60 minutes or until bubbling and golden brown. Cool 30 minutes to thicken before serving.

Serve warm with a scoop of dairy-free vanilla ice cream or vegan whipped cream.

Variations
Substitute blackberries for a blend of blueberries, raspberries and strawberries. For tart fruits like blueberries, increase sugar to 1/3 cup.

To increase the fiber content, add 2 tablespoons ground flaxseed to the flour mixture.

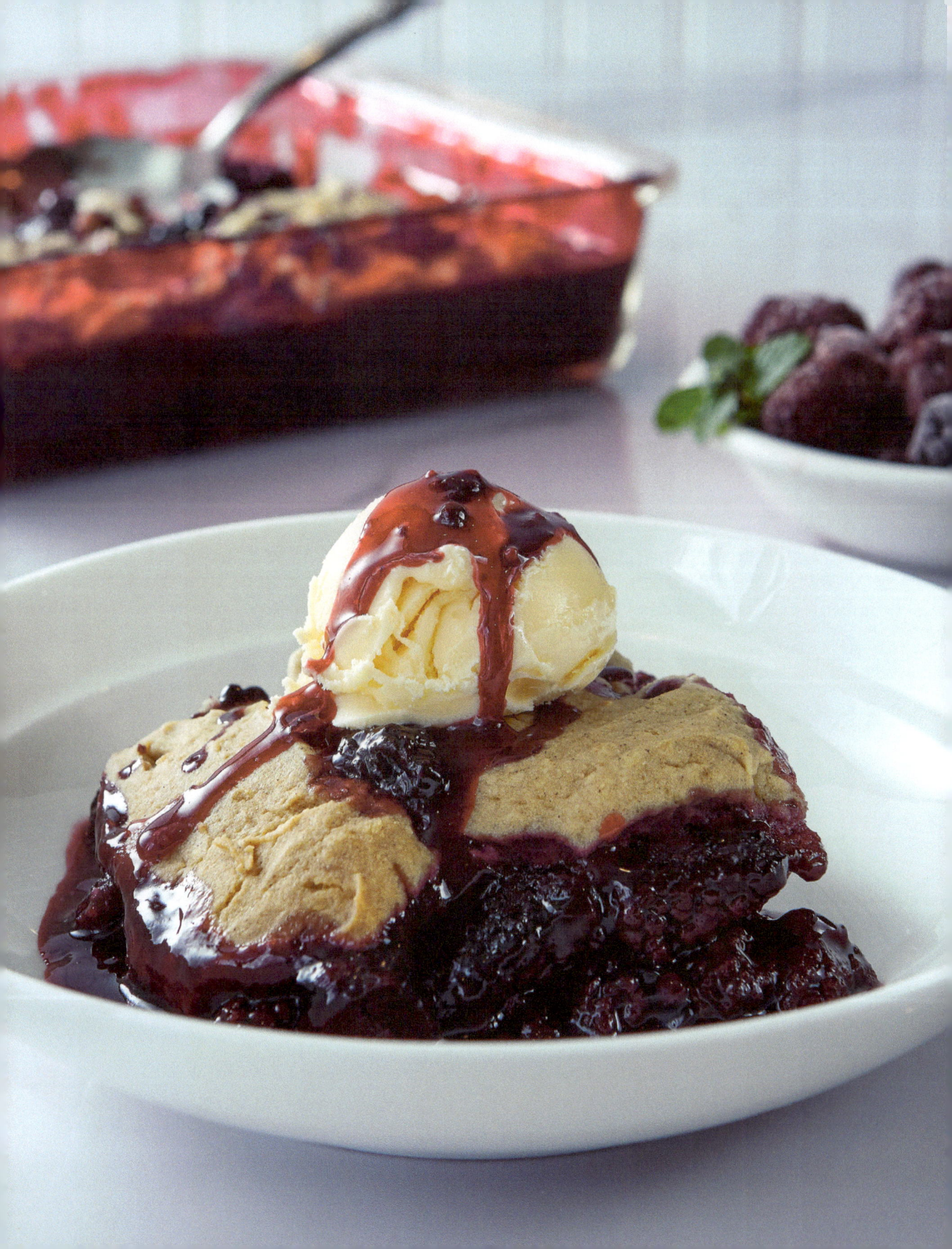

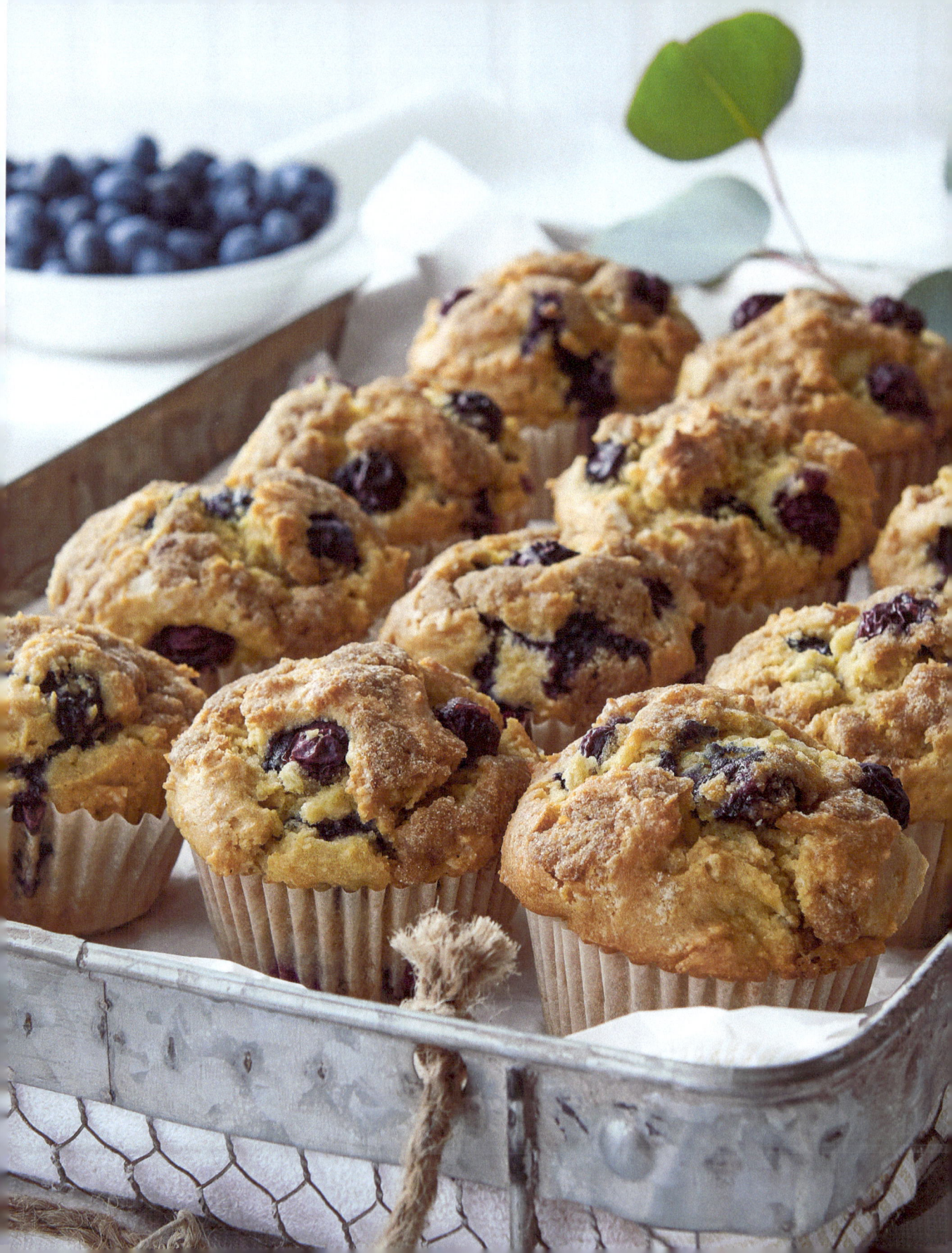

Blueberry Muffins

prep time	bake time	yield
10 minutes	**25 minutes**	**12 muffins**

Psst! The secret to a fluffy and tender muffin is to keep the butter crumb frozen. Soft butter will make them dense. Whether you enjoy them for breakfast or as a cozy afternoon treat, they offer the perfect balance of sweet and tangy that will brighten your day.

Equipment: Stand mixer with paddle attachment

Preheat oven to 375 degrees F. Line a muffin tin with paper cups.

In a small bowl, stir milk and apple cider vinegar. Set aside.

In the stand mixer bowl with paddle attachment, whisk flour blend, almond flour, sugar, baking powder, baking soda, lemon zest and salt. Add butter cubes and beat on low to medium until the mixture resembles a crumb with pea-sized pieces of butter.

In a medium bowl, whisk milk mixture, eggs, sourdough starter and lemon juice.

Add milk mixture to the flour mixture. Combine on low for 30 seconds. Scrape clean the sides of the bowl. Mix again for 30 seconds. The mixture will be thick. Do not over mix.

Gently fold in blueberries using a rubber spatula.

Fill paper cups to the top with batter. Sprinkle generously with streusel topping.

Bake 25 minutes until tops are golden brown. Remove to a wire rack to cool completely.

Streusel Topping

Combine butter, brown sugar and flour blend in a small bowl. Sprinkle atop muffins before baking.

Use fresh or frozen blueberries with delicious results.

1/2 cup milk alternative

1 tablespoon apple cider vinegar

2 cups gluten-free flour blend

1 cup almond flour

1/2 cup sugar

2 teaspoons baking powder

1 teaspoon baking soda

1 teaspoon fresh lemon zest

1/2 teaspoon salt

1/2 cup (1 stick) vegan butter, diced and frozen

2 eggs, beaten

1/3 cup gluten-free sourdough starter

2 tablespoons fresh lemon juice

1 cup blueberries

Streusel Topping

3 tablespoons vegan butter, soft

3 tablespoons brown sugar

1 tablespoon of gluten-free flour blend

Chocolate Bundt Cake

prep time	bake time	yield
10 minutes	**45 minutes**	**10-inch bundt cake**

Chocolate oozes a tenacious attraction. Paired with the charming shape of a bundt pan and what's not to love? This recipe for a full-size cake can be divided into adorable mini bundts as well. The coffee in this version enhances the rich chocolate flavor. The sourdough starter adds scrumptious moisture to each bite. Make this impressive cake for your next celebration at home or potluck, I promise no one will know it's gluten-free!

Equipment: Stand mixer with paddle attachment

1/2 cup (1 stick) vegan butter

1/2 cup sugar

2 eggs, beaten

1 cup gluten-free sourdough starter

1/2 cup strong coffee, cooled

1/4 cup milk alternative

1 teaspoon vanilla

2 cups gluten-free flour blend

1/2 cup cocoa powder

2 teaspoons baking powder

1 teaspoon baking soda

1 teaspoon salt

1/2 cup dairy-free chocolate chips

Ganache

1/4 cup dairy free chocolate chips

1 to 2 tablespoons milk alternative

Preheat the oven to 350 degrees F. Butter bundt pan and dust lightly with flour blend or cocoa powder.

In a stand mixer with paddle attachment, cream butter and sugar until fluffy. Add eggs, sourdough starter, coffee, milk and vanilla. Mix on low for 30 seconds. Scrape clean the sides of the bowl. Mix again until combined.

In a separate medium bowl, whisk together flour blend, cocoa powder, baking powder, baking soda and salt.

Add flour mixture to the sugar mixture. Mix on low then increase speed to combine thoroughly. Mixture will be fluffy and thick. Stir in chocolate chips.

Pour evenly into prepared bundt pan. Gently tap pan on the counter to allow any bubbles to compact and smooth out the top.

Bake 45 minutes or until a toothpick comes out clean when tested in the center. Do not overbake. Cool in the pan 20 minutes then invert on a wire rack. Drizzle with chocolate ganache. Cool completely before slicing.

Ganache

In a small microwave safe bowl, microwave chocolate chips and milk on 60 percent power for 30 seconds then stir.

Repeat heating and stirring until smooth and chocolate will drizzle in a solid stream off a spoon. Drizzle atop warm cake as desired.

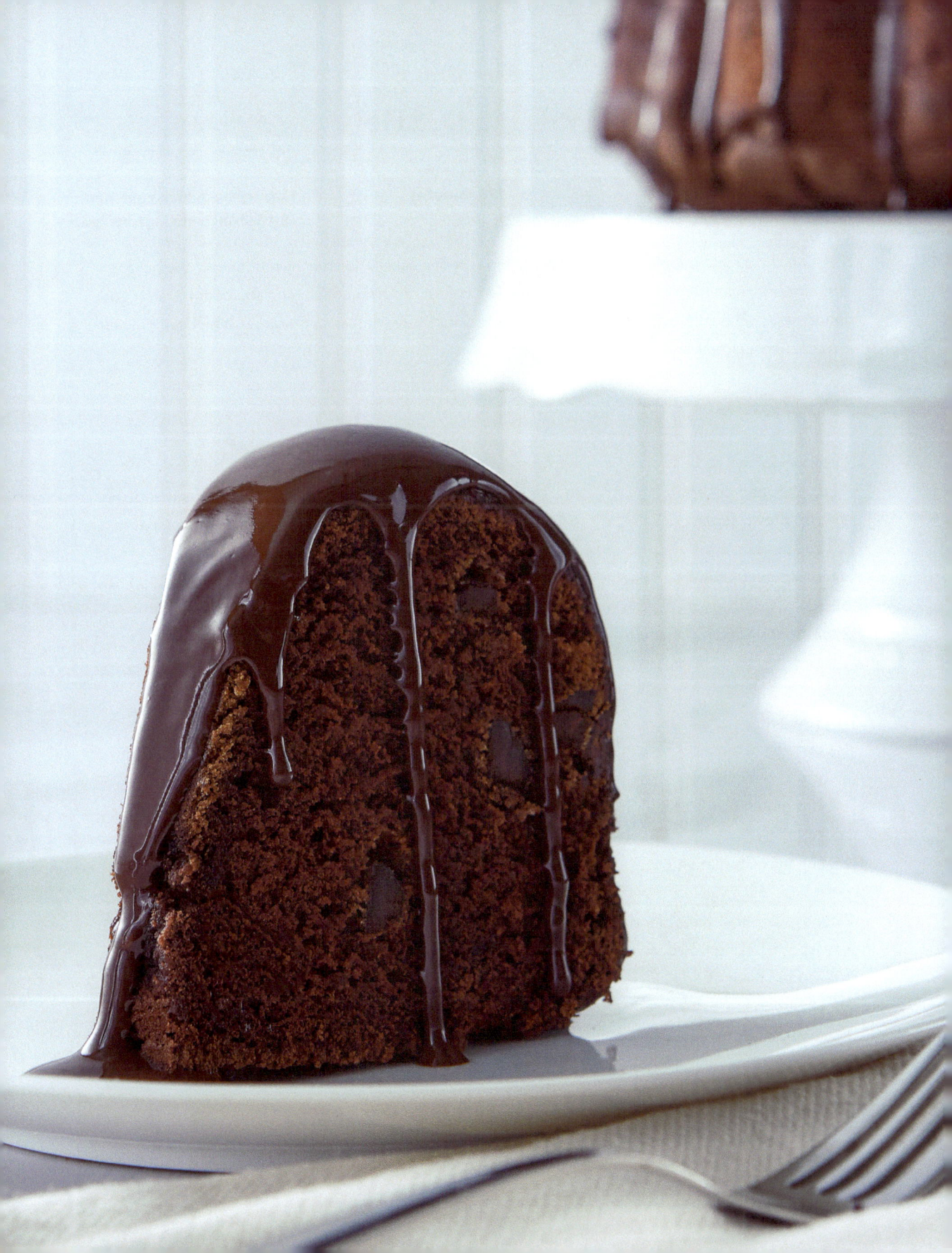

Coffee Cake with Pecans

prep time	bake time	yield
20 minutes	**30 minutes**	**13-by-9-by-3-inch cake pan or 9-by-3-inch springform pan**

The only thing most people like more than coffee is coffee cake! The crunchy nuttiness of the pecans and hint of cinnamon make it a perfect companion to your morning coffee. The sourdough starter adds tenderness to the crumb and a faint tang that enhances the sweetness of the sugar. It's a beautiful balance that pleases a crowd any time of day.

Equipment: Stand mixer with paddle attachment

Pecan topping

1 cup chopped pecans

3/4 cup brown sugar, packed

1/4 cup vegan butter

1 tablespoon gluten-free flour blend

2 teaspoons Ceylon cinnamon

Cake

1 cup sugar

1/2 cup vegan butter

3 eggs

1/2 cup gluten-free sourdough starter

1/4 cup milk alternative

2 cups gluten-free flour blend

1 teaspoon baking powder

1 teaspoon baking soda

1/2 teaspoon salt

1 cup vegan sour cream or plain vegan yogurt

3/4 cup raisins, rehydrated in hot water 10 minutes, drained

Pecan topping

In a small bowl with a fork, stir brown sugar, flour blend and cinnamon. Cut in butter with a fork to make a crumble mixture. Stir in chopped pecans. Set aside.

Cake

Preheat oven to 350 degrees F. Lightly butter cake pan.

In a stand mixer with paddle attachment, cream sugar and butter until fluffy. Add eggs, sourdough starter and milk. Mix on low to combine.

In a separate medium bowl, whisk flour blend, baking powder, baking soda and salt.

Add the flour mixture to the butter mixture. Combine on low. Fold in raisins and sour cream by hand.

Spread into prepared baking pan. Sprinkle evenly with pecan topping. Bake 30 minutes or until a toothpick tested in the center comes out clean.

Serve warm or set on wire rack to cool in the pan.

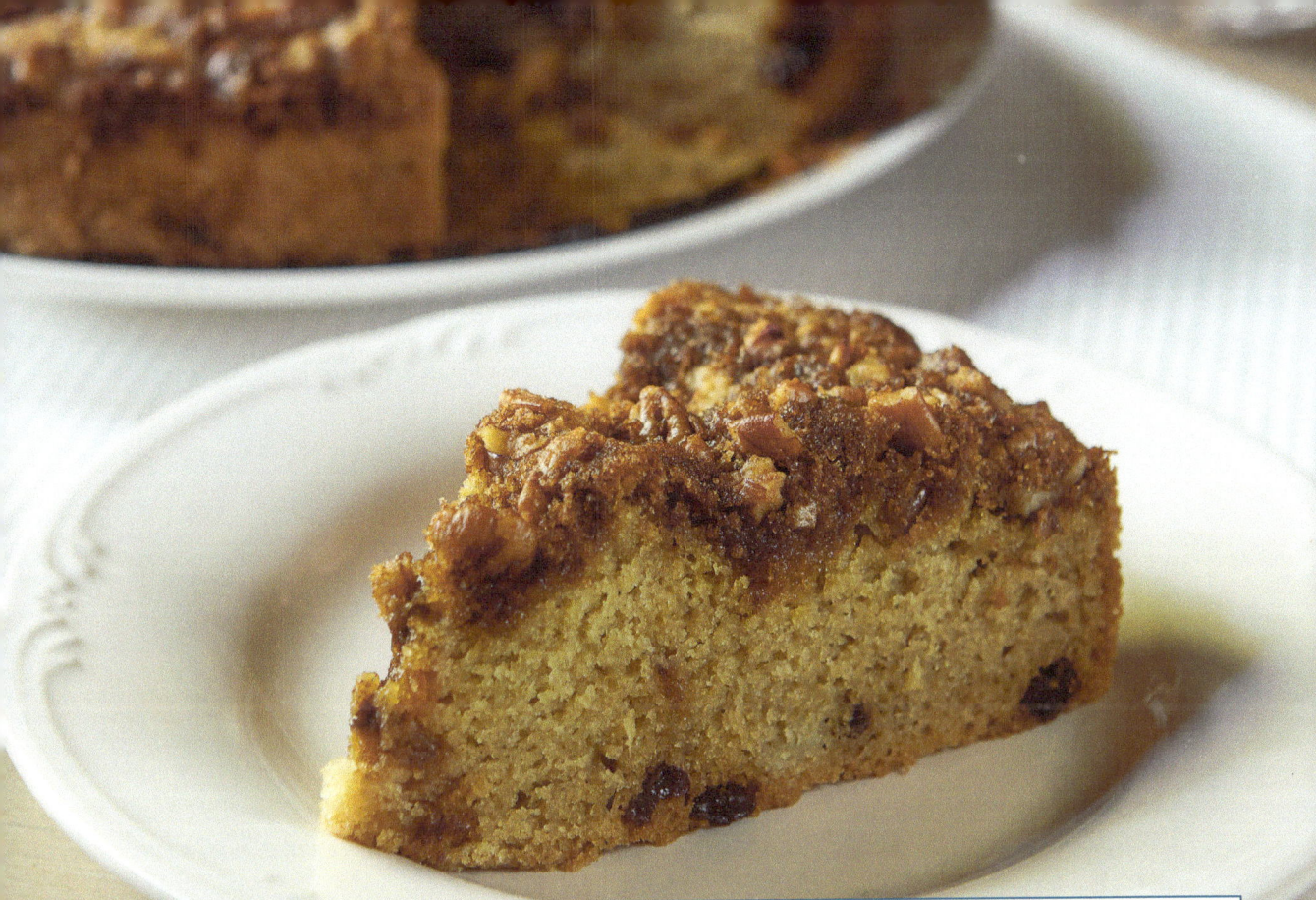

Brown Sugar

yield
2 cups

Molasses is a kitchen staple that, like honey, never seems to go bad and is handy to keep in the pantry. Once you make your own brown sugar, you'll never buy it again.

Equipment: Stand mixer with paddle attachment

In a stand mixer with paddle attachment, combine sugar and molasses until completely combined, about 2 minutes. Scrape the sides and bottom of the bowl and mix until blended.
Adjust the amount of molasses depending on the level of light or dark brown sugar desired. The ratio of this recipe makes a medium to dark brown sugar that works perfectly for recipes in this cookbook.
Store in airtight container. This brown sugar will not get hard or dry like store-bought brown sugar.

2 cups granulated sugar
1 1/2 tablespoons molasses

Crepes

prep time	bake time	yield
5 minutes plus	**5 to 8 minutes each**	**6 10-inch crepes**
30 minutes rest		

Unlock your inner Parisian chef with these tender but sturdy crepes! With countless topping and filling options, they are perfect for an easy dinner or a scrumptious dessert. I'm convinced this is the tastiest way to use sourdough discard. A specialized crepe pan or tools are not needed! I have used 10-inch stainless steel and ceramic skillets with success.

2 eggs, beaten

1 1/2 cup milk alternative, plus more as needed

2 tablespoons vegan butter, melted

2 tablespoons gluten-free sourdough starter

3 tablespoons superfine sugar, omit for a savory crepe

1 1/2 cups gluten-free flour blend

1 teaspoon baking powder

Butter or oil for skillet

In a medium mixing bowl, combine eggs, milk, butter, starter and sugar if using. Add flour blend and baking powder. Stir into a smooth and thin batter. Add more milk to thin, as needed. If using a whisk, be careful not to whip the egg whites.

Rest for 30 minutes to hydrate the flours. Batter may be covered and refrigerated overnight.

Heat skillet on medium-high to mercury ball stage, when a 1/8 teaspoon of water forms a rolling ball when added. Butter skillet with 1/2 to 1 tablespoon vegan butter. Pour 1/2 cup batter into skillet. Working quickly, tilt and swirl batter into a thin, even layer. For 10-inch skillet, 1/2 cup of batter will generously fill the pan. Melt more butter in skillet before each crepe.

Cook until crepe bubbles emerge and burst across the surface, 3 to 4 minutes. The underside should be a rich golden brown then flip. Add toppings, fold in half or quarters. Serve warm.

Variations

Savory crepe

Add 1/2 teaspoon freshly minced rosemary or your favorite herb to batter. Top with prosciutto and vegan mozzarella.

Sweet crepe

Top with honey, Ceylon cinnamon and vegan butter, or fill with diced fruit and drizzle with heated almond butter.

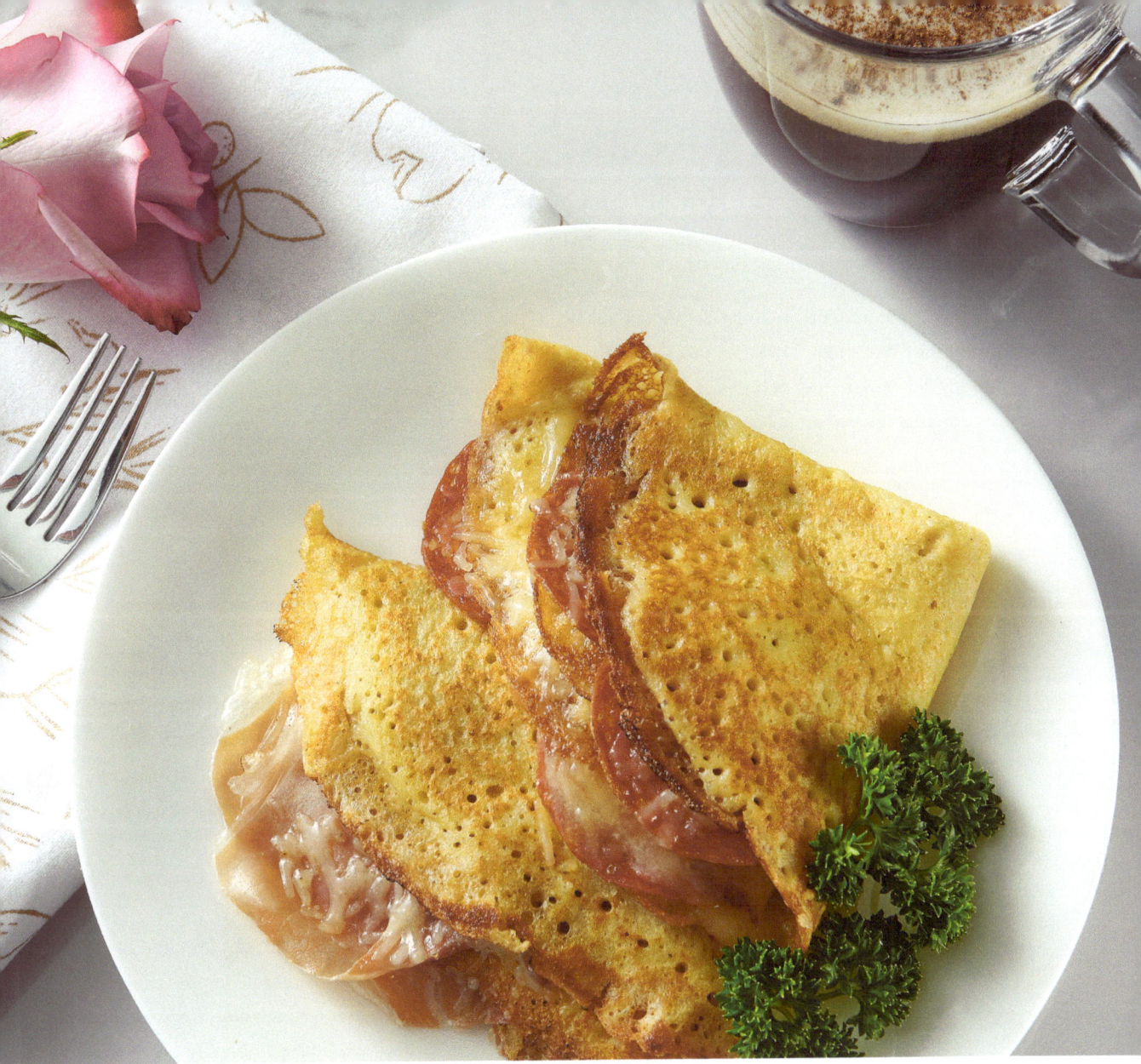

Superfine Sugar

Add 2 cups granulated sugar to a food processor.
Cover the blending bowl with a clean towel to contain dust. Pulse until the sugar crystals are very fine, about 30 seconds.

Lemon Pound Cake

prep time	bake time	yield
15 minutes	**90 minutes**	**9-by-4-inch Pullman loaf**

I'll be the first to admit that lemon desserts aren't usually my jam. I whip up lemon bars for my husband, knowing they won't tempt me! But this gluten-free sourdough lemon pound cake has changed the game – it's subtly flavored, tender and sweet, making it a delightful treat I can't resist. With the extra zesty lemon drizzle on top, it's perfect for those who love a citrusy twist!

Equipment: Stand mixer with paddle attachment

6 tablespoons (3/4 stick) vegan butter, soft
1/2 cup sugar
2 eggs, beaten
1 cup gluten-free sourdough starter
1/4 cup milk alternative
Juice of 2 medium lemons (1/3 to 1/2 cup)
1 teaspoon vanilla

2 cups gluten-free flour blend
1/2 cup almond flour
Zest of 2 medium lemons (1 to 2 tablespoons lightly packed)
2 teaspoons baking powder
1 teaspoon baking soda
1 teaspoon salt

Lemon Drizzle
1/2 cup powdered sugar
2 tablespoons fresh lemon juice
Zest of 1 lemon

Preheat oven to 350 degrees F. Lightly butter loaf pan.

In a stand mixer with paddle attachment, cream butter and sugar. Add eggs, starter, milk, lemon juice, vanilla and poppyseeds* if using. Mix on low to combine, scrape clean the sides of the bowl.

In a separate medium bowl, whisk flour blend, almond flour, lemon zest, baking powder, baking soda and salt. Add flour mixture to the butter mixture. Mix on low for 30 seconds. Increase to medium speed until combined, about 1 minute. Mixture will be fluffy and thick. Stir in bluberries* if using.

Pour into prepared loaf pan. Draw a deep line down the center of the batter.

Bake 90 minutes or until a toothpick comes out clean from the center. Loosely tent with foil if crust browns before internal temperature reaches 210 degrees F. Cool in the pan for 20 minutes. Remove from pan and apply lemon drizzle as desired. Cool completely a wire rack before slicing.

Lemon Drizzle

In a small bowl, stir sugar, lemon juice and zest to combine thoroughly. Drizzle generously atop warm cake.

*Try adding 1 tablespoon poppyseeds or 1/2 cup fresh blueberries for a fun twist!

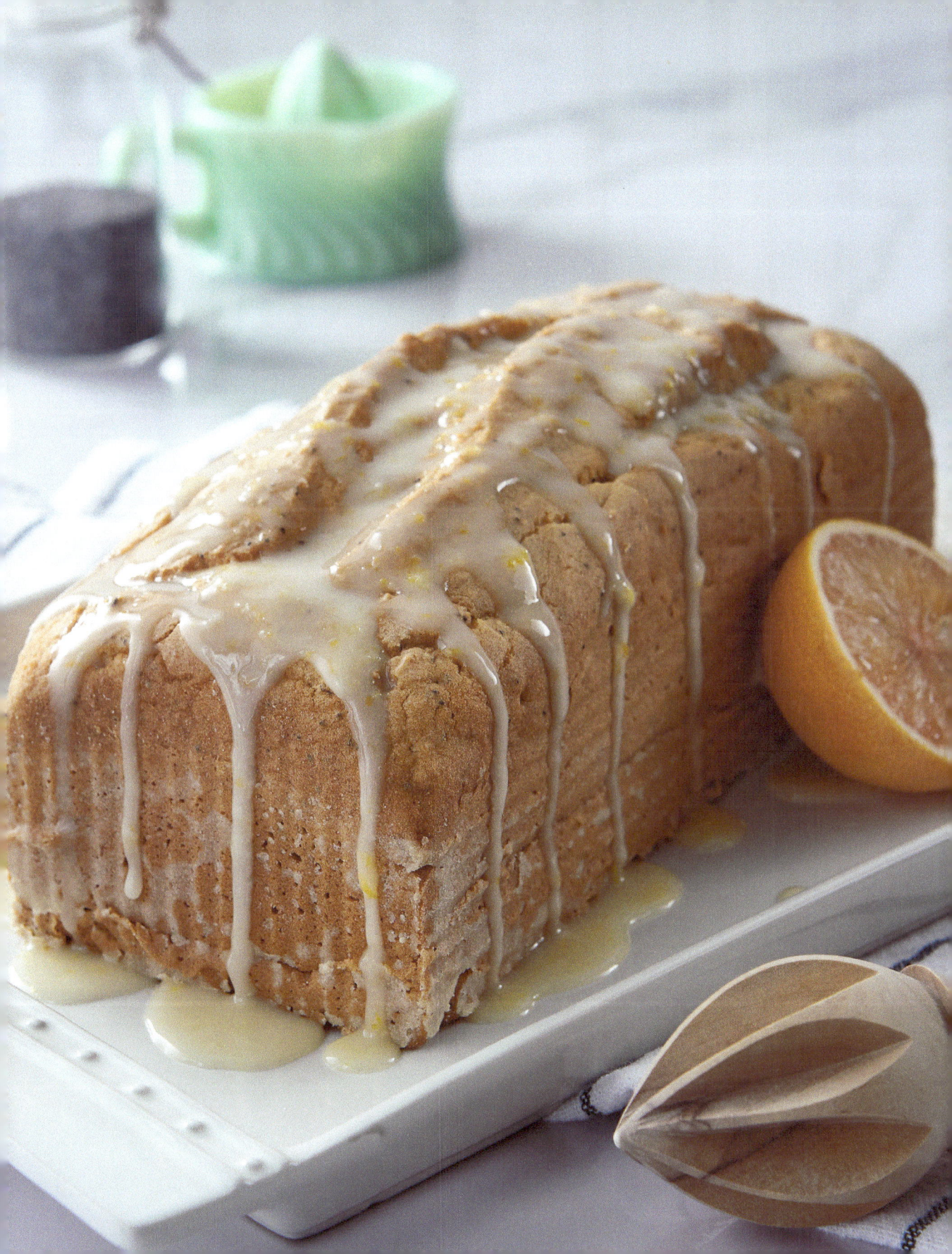

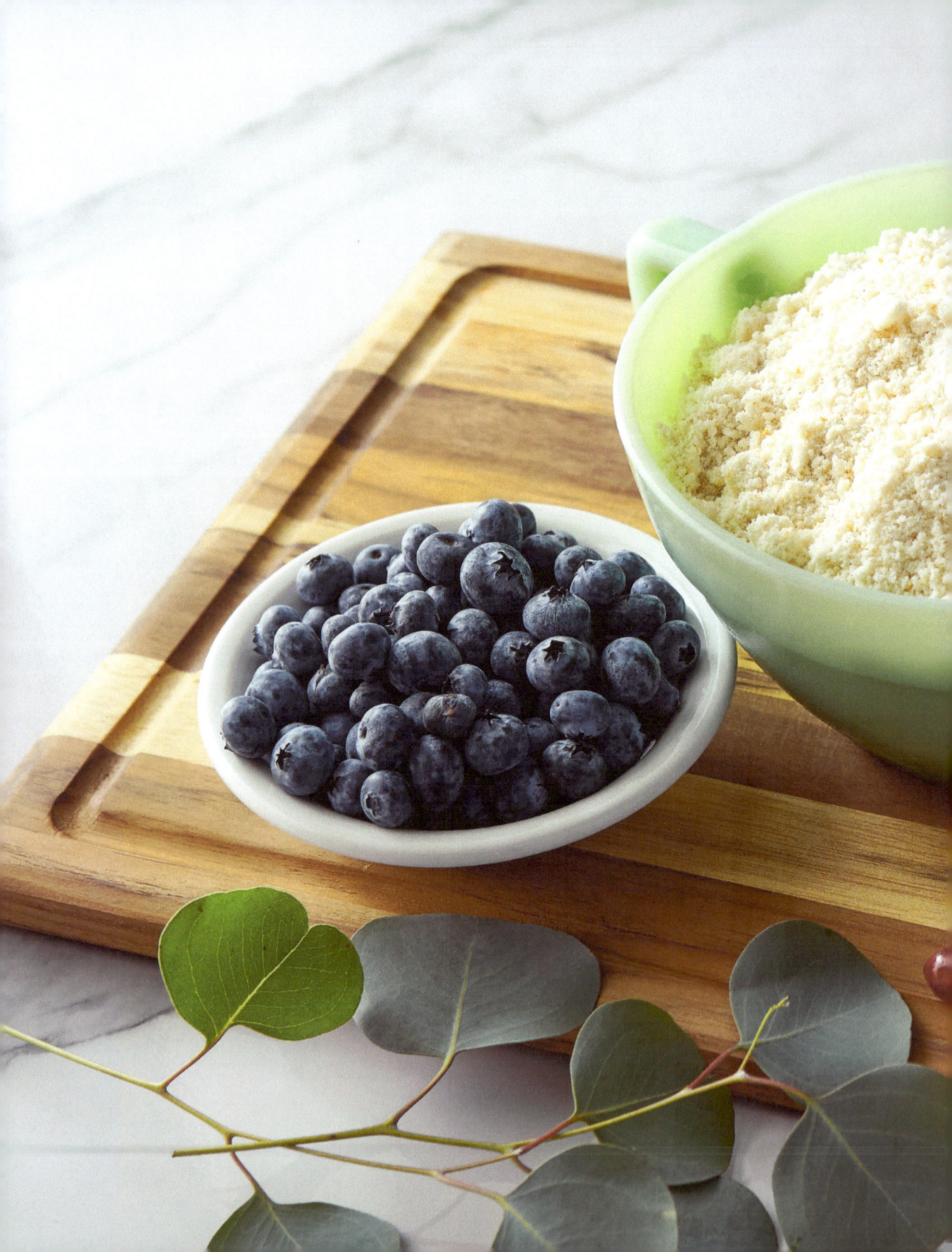

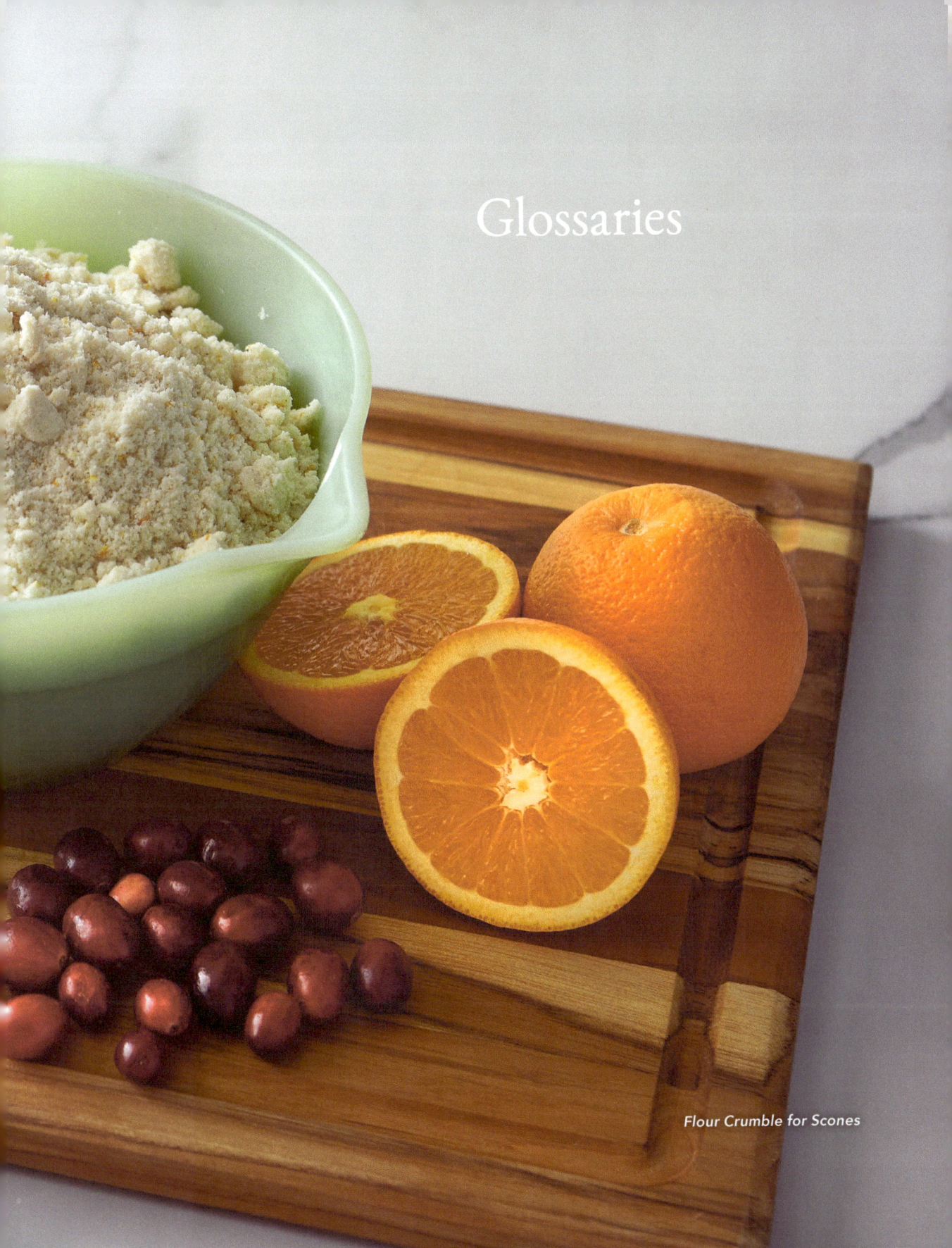

Glossaries

Flour Crumble for Scones

How to Read Ingredients List

Pay particular attention to the *placement* of a description or action for the ingredient.

If the action is listed **before** the ingredient, perform the action then measure.

1/2 cup **chopped** nuts
Chop the nuts *then* measure them

1 cup **sifted** gluten-free flour blend
Sift flour *then* measure 1 cup of the sifted flour using the Scoop-and-Sweep method

1 cup **stirred** full-fat, unsweetened coconut milk
Stir full-fat, unsweetened coconut milk *then* measure 1 cup

If the action is listed **after** the ingredient, measure the ingredient then perform the action.

1/2 cup raisins, **rehydrated** in hot water 10 minutes, drained
Measure dry raisins *then* rehydrate in boiling hot water for 10 minutes, drain all the water before adding to the recipe

1 cup gluten-free flour blend, **sifted**
Measure 1 cup flour using the Scoop-and-Sweep method *then* sift and use whole amount

1/2 cup brown sugar, **packed**
Firmly press brown sugar into 1/2 cup, level-off, *then* add to recipe

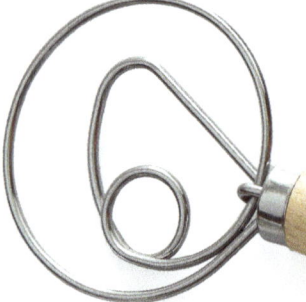

Dutch Dough Hook

Kitchen and Pantry Guide

Special tools and equipment used often

Active Dry Yeast

Danish dough hook, whisk or sturdy rubber spatula

Dutch oven with oven-safe lid

Food processor with dough blade

Milk alternative (unsweetened and unflavored oat or almond milk)

Popover pan (deep and steep-sided cupcake pan)

Pullman loaf pan (9-by-4-inch)

Silicone baking mat

Stand mixer with paddle and dough hook attachments

Unbleached parchment paper

Products frequently used in this book

Baking powder

Bee's Wrap® resusable beeswax wrap

Bob's Red Mill Gluten-Free 1-to-1 Baking Flour Blend

County Crock plant butter

Fine crystal sea salt

Ground flax meal

Local honey

Nutritional yeast

One Degree Organics Gluten-Free Sprouted Rolled Oats

Sorghum flour

Kitchen environment

Keeping a clean kitchen is important for maintaining a healthy gluten-free sourdough starter. Examine your kitchen cleaning products. Products containing bleach are too harsh to support healthy sourdough starter. Commercial disinfectant sprays disperse into the air which can affect the growth and vigor of your sourdough starter. Look for an all-natural cleaner or make your own with this recipe.

Homemade orange vinegar

Orange peels are not beneficial for the compost heap and chickens won't eat them, but don't throw them away! Use them to make your own orange vinegar.

As you use oranges, slice most of the white pith from the peels leaving a thick layer of fragrant, oily orange zest. Place peels in a sealed container of 5% white vinegar. Set aside to rest for 2 months or longer to allow the oil to infuse into the vinegar. Shake container once a week. Vinegar will take on a deep orange color when ready to use.

Kitchen counter cleaner

Combine equal parts homemade orange vinegar,* rubbing alcohol and filtered water with 3 to 5 drops of your favorite essential oil(s) for scent.

Use 5 to 10 drops of orange essential oil in white vinegar until you have homemade orange vinegar.

Kitchen Thermometers

Every kitchen needs three different thermometers. In my cooking classes, students often ask how we know when a food is properly cooked and safe to eat. My answer usually includes using a thermometer. Purchase the proper type of thermometer depending on its intended use.

1. Refrigerator thermometer

Refrigerator temperature should range between 35 and 40 degrees F. Equip your refrigerator with a refrigerator thermometer to ensure the temperature is safely in this range. If above 40 degrees F, bacterial growth in foods will accelerate. This can spell disaster for breeding bad bacteria and ruin your sourdough starter. If below 32 degrees F, your foods will freeze. Luckily, freezing sourdough starter does not typically spell disaster. Simply, thaw and feed. See **Starter Care**.

2. Oven thermometer

Ovens are designed to cycle temperature, typically fluctuating 25 degrees F above and below the set temperature. To ensure your breads bake properly, use an oven thermometer and always set a timer – relying on visual clues alone can lead you to thinking bread is done when it is not.

3. Food thermometer

The internal temperature of breads should reach at least 210 degrees F. Keep in mind that some gluten-free bread recipes may require additional time after reaching this temperature to avoid gumminess.

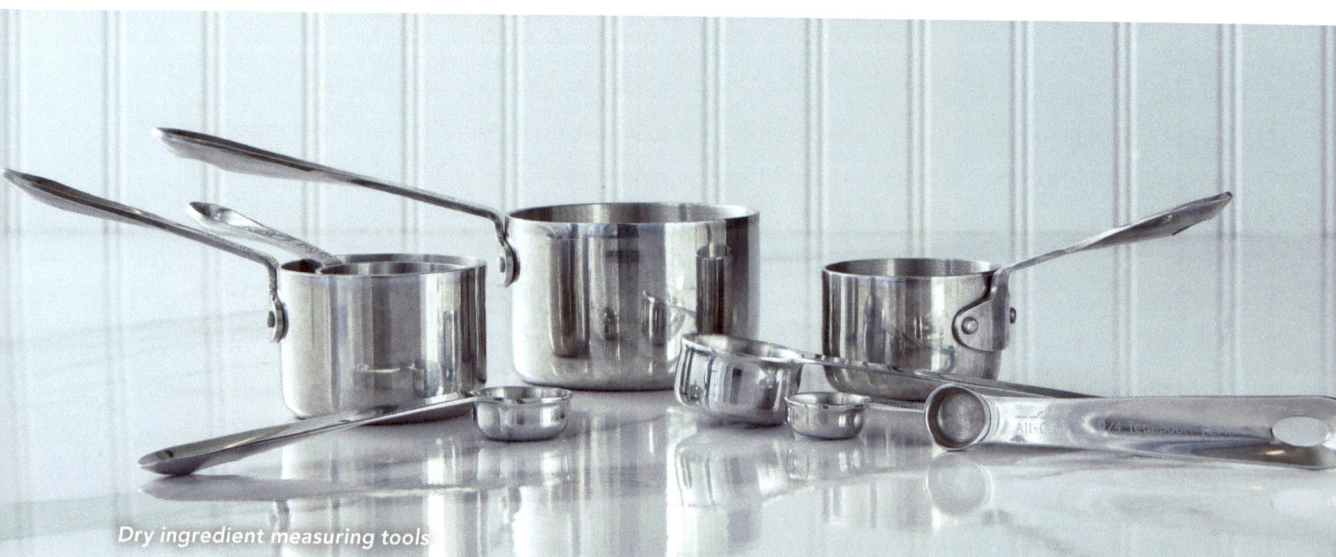

Dry ingredient measuring tools

Measuring Tools

Moisture balance can be tricky with gluten-free sourdough baking, making it essential to use the correct measuring tools.

Liquid ingredient measuring tools
Measure liquids with graduated liquid measuring cups.

Dry ingredient measuring tools
Measure dry ingredients such as flour blends, oats, salt, cinnamon, seeds and nuts in graduated dry measuring cups and spoons.

Dash or pinch = 1/8 teaspoon

1 1/2 teaspoon = 1/2 tablespoon

3 teaspoons = 1 tablespoon

2 tablespoons = 1/8 cup

4 tablespoons = 1/4 cup

6 tablespoons = 1/3 cup

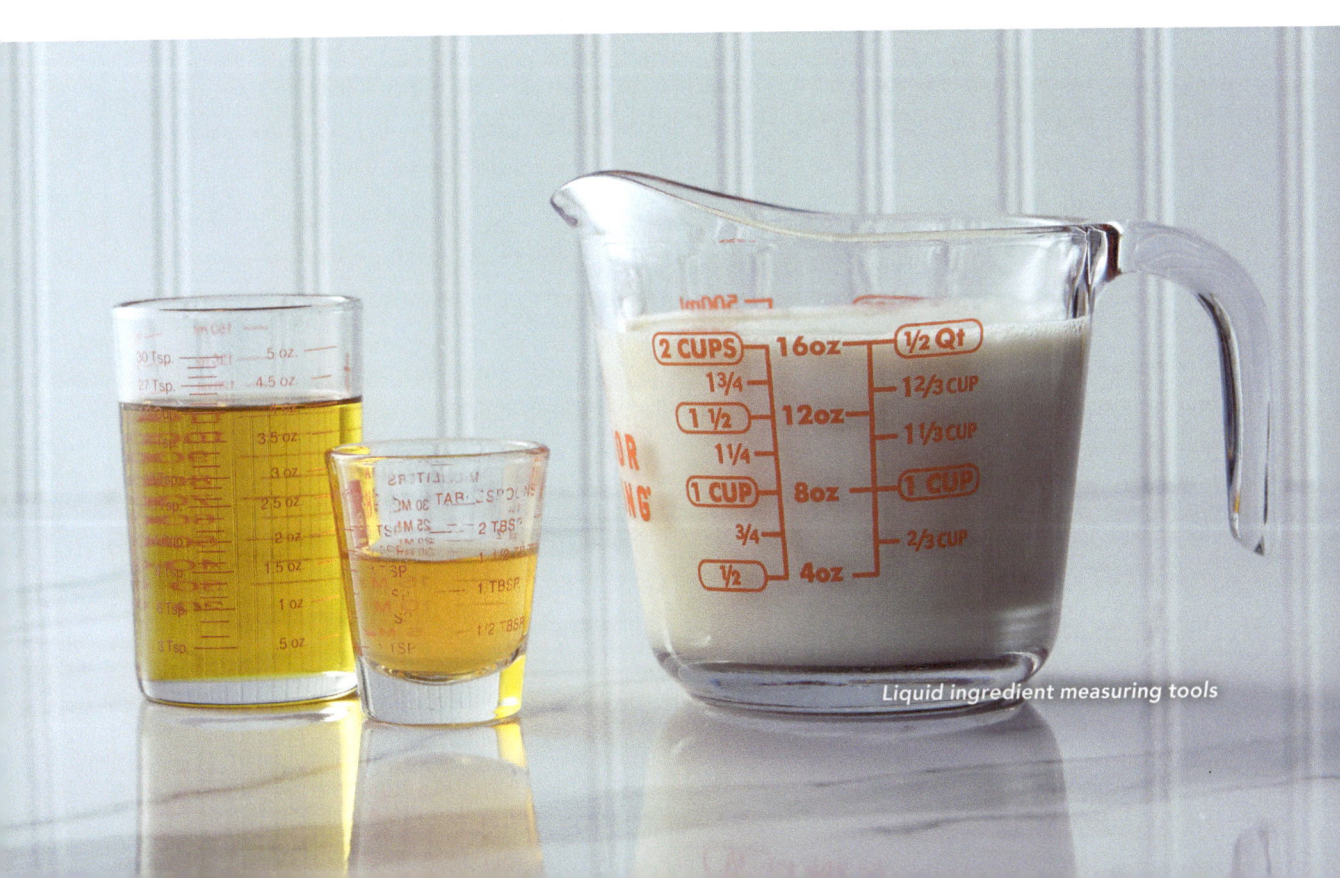

Liquid ingredient measuring tools

Gluten-Free Flours

Arrowroot
A finely ground powder made from the root of a South American plant. It's often used as a substitute for cornstarch to thicken sauces. While low in nutritional value, arrowroot flour helps lighten the texture of baked goods when combined with other flours.

Buckwheat
Despite its name, buckwheat flour is not related to wheat. Made from ground buckwheat groats, it's high in protein and has a slightly nutty flavor. Buckwheat flour adds moisture and tenderness to baked goods. When substituting it, you may need to reduce the liquid in the recipe. Its dense, chewy texture makes it perfect in baguettes.

Brown rice
More nutrient-dense than white rice flour, brown rice flour has a nutty, toasted flavor. It works well in muffins, as a thickener for soups, or as a breading for fried foods. Brown rice flour can also be milled at home using a high-power food processor.

Chickpea
Chickpea flour is ideal for recipes that don't need much rise, like flatbreads or pizza crusts. It has a mild, beany flavor that can be mellowed by toasting the flour before use or by blending it with other gluten-free flours.

Coconut
Coconut flour is highly absorbent and works best in recipes with high moisture content. If used in excess, it can make baked goods dry and gritty. Coconut flour pairs best in small quantities or with bold flavors. Avoid using it in recipes requiring leavening, as its heaviness affects the rise.

Millet
Available in dark, white and yellow varieties, millet flour has different antioxidant properties depending on the type. One of the oldest grains still cultivated today, pearl millet is the most widely grown variety and is high in iron. With a mild flavor and high protein content, millet flour is great for making your own gluten-free flour blend.

Sorghum
A versatile, nutrient-rich flour with a smooth texture and mild flavor, sorghum (also known as great millet or jowar) contains no lectins, making it easier to digest. High in protein, it's commonly used in cakes, breads and many other baked goods.

Tapioca
Made from the cassava root, tapioca flour is prized for its high starch content, which adds elasticity to baked goods. It's commonly used as a thickener, like cornstarch, or combined with other flours to provide structure and chew. Limit volume of tapioca flour and pair it with fiber to help stabilize impact on blood sugar.

Types of Gluten-Free Flours

Neutral flours
- brown rice flour
- sorghum flour
- sweet rice flour
- white rice flour

High-protein flour
- amaranth flour
- buckwheat flour
- chickpea flour
- millet flour
- oat flour
- quinoa flour
- sorghum flour

High-fiber flour
- amaranth flour
- buckwheat flour
- chickpea flour
- oat flour
- quinoa flour

Stabilizer
- ground flax seed
- ground chia seed
- potato flour (not potato starch)

Starches
- arrowroot powder
- cornstarch
- potato starch (not potato flour)
- sweet potato flour
- tapioca starch (also called tapioca flour)

Gums
- agar powder
- whole psyllium husk powder
- xanthan gum

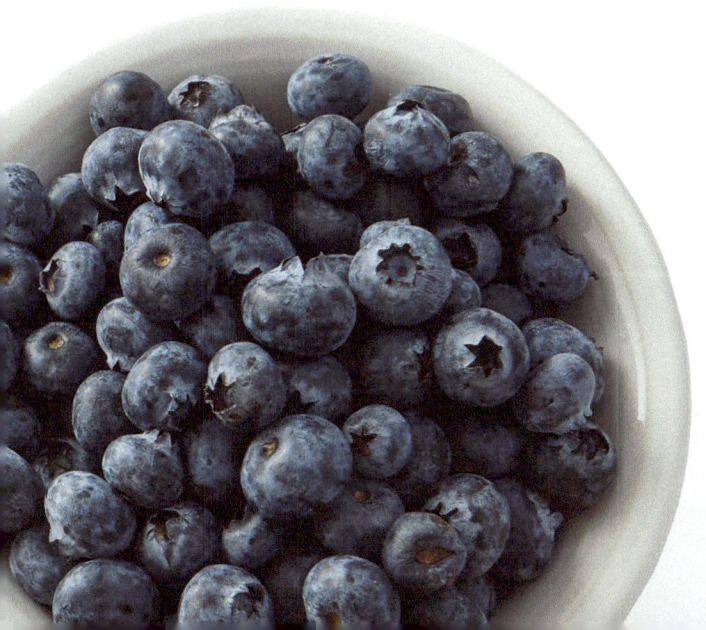

Conversions and Substitutions

As you become familiar with gluten-free recipes and techniques, the following tips will help you make these recipes your own. It can take a few tries to get proportions just right when substituting gluten-free flour blends, but with practice, you'll find what works best. **Foundations of Baking Gluten-Free Sourdough** (p. 18), **Glossary of Gluten-Free Flours** and this section work together to guide you toward success.

For example, brown rice flour can be used instead of Bob's Red Mill Gluten-Free 1-to-1 Baking Flour to grow and feed your starter. You can make your own by grinding organic whole-grain brown rice in a grain mill or high-speed blender until very fine. However, feeding long-term with a single flour like brown rice will result in a less resilient starter. If you're new to gluten-free sourdough starter, it's best to start with the recommended Bob's Gluten-Free blend, then experiment with making your own flour blend once you're familiar with sourdough starter care.

Gluten-free flour blend example
>   2 parts brown rice flour
>   2 parts sorghum or millet flour
>   1 part cornstarch or tapioca starch

Add whole psyllium husk powder as 1:1 substitution for xanthan gum

Active Dry Yeast vs Instant Dry Yeast
>   Active Dry Yeast is often activated, or *proofed*, before use, while Instant Dry Yeast is used directly from the package. Most recipes in this cookbook call for Active Dry Yeast with a proofing step. I prefer this method because it allows you to see the yeast in action, giving you confidence that your dough will rise beautifully.

Replace dry yeast with sourdough starter in any recipe
>   A good starting point is to replace 1 teaspoon of dry active yeast with 1/2 cup of active starter and reduce flour by 1/3 cup and liquids by a total of 1/3 cup.

Egg substitutions
>   1 egg: 1 tablespoon ground flax seeds or chia seeds dissolved in 3 tablespoons warm water

Acknowledgments

It feels nothing short of miraculous to work with true professionals like Rae and Jason. What were the odds? I set out to create a one-of-a-kind cookbook and two exceptionally talented individuals – a graphic designer and a food photographer – just happened to be right at my doorstep. With the support of an incredible network of people, this cookbook took shape in just six months! To say I lucked out is an understatement – I'm truly blessed.

Special thank you to **Rae Zurcher**, a brilliant designer and the most refreshingly kind and honest taste-tester. Rae's sharp eye and boundless creativity brought this beautiful book to life.
Thank you to **Jason Gamble**, an extraordinary food photographer and the hardest worker I know. Jason's dedication to excellence of his craft shines through in every shot, every edit and every deadline exceeded.

I don't think this book would have taken shape without my dietetic intern, **Myesha Thomas**. Thank you for your kindness, humor and help. Myesha has been cooking alongside me since she was in sixth grade! It's been an honor to be her mentor on her road to becoming a registered dietitian.
A warm thank you to **Maggie Green**, cookbook writing coach and culinary dietitian, for keeping all my ideas on track. Without your guidance, this cookbook would still be stuck in my notebooks and binders.

To my husband, **Kelly Lobb MD** – thank you for being my biggest supporter, my patient recipe tester and my most forgiving food critic. Your unwavering love and belief in me make me believe I can accomplish anything.
To my daughter, **Caroline**, who always had wise words and pep talks to help me push through writer's block and the self-doubt of starting this new chapter of my career.
To my son, **Jack**, whose humor lifted my spirits through many recipe fails. Extra kudos to you for eating gluten- and dairy-free with grace and very few complaints.
Thank you to my Mimi, **Frances Lobb**. Never has there been such a darling and supportive mother-in-law. I admire your optimism and adore you for your endless encouragement.
Thank you to **Ruth Gamble**, whose high praise of my gluten-free breads planted the seeds of possibility in my kitchen experiments, which ultimately became this cookbook.

A big thank you to my family and friends for bravely eating my recipes – flops and all! Gluten-free recipe development often means gooey cakes and gummy or rock-hard loaves of bread. And a shout out to my recipe testers! You were all invaluable to making sure these recipes got translated properly out of my head and are successful as written.

And finally, thanks to **Bob's Red Mill**, **Bee's Wrap®** and to **One Degree Organics** for generously providing samples and products for recipe development, recipe testers and students of Appetite to Travel cooking classes.

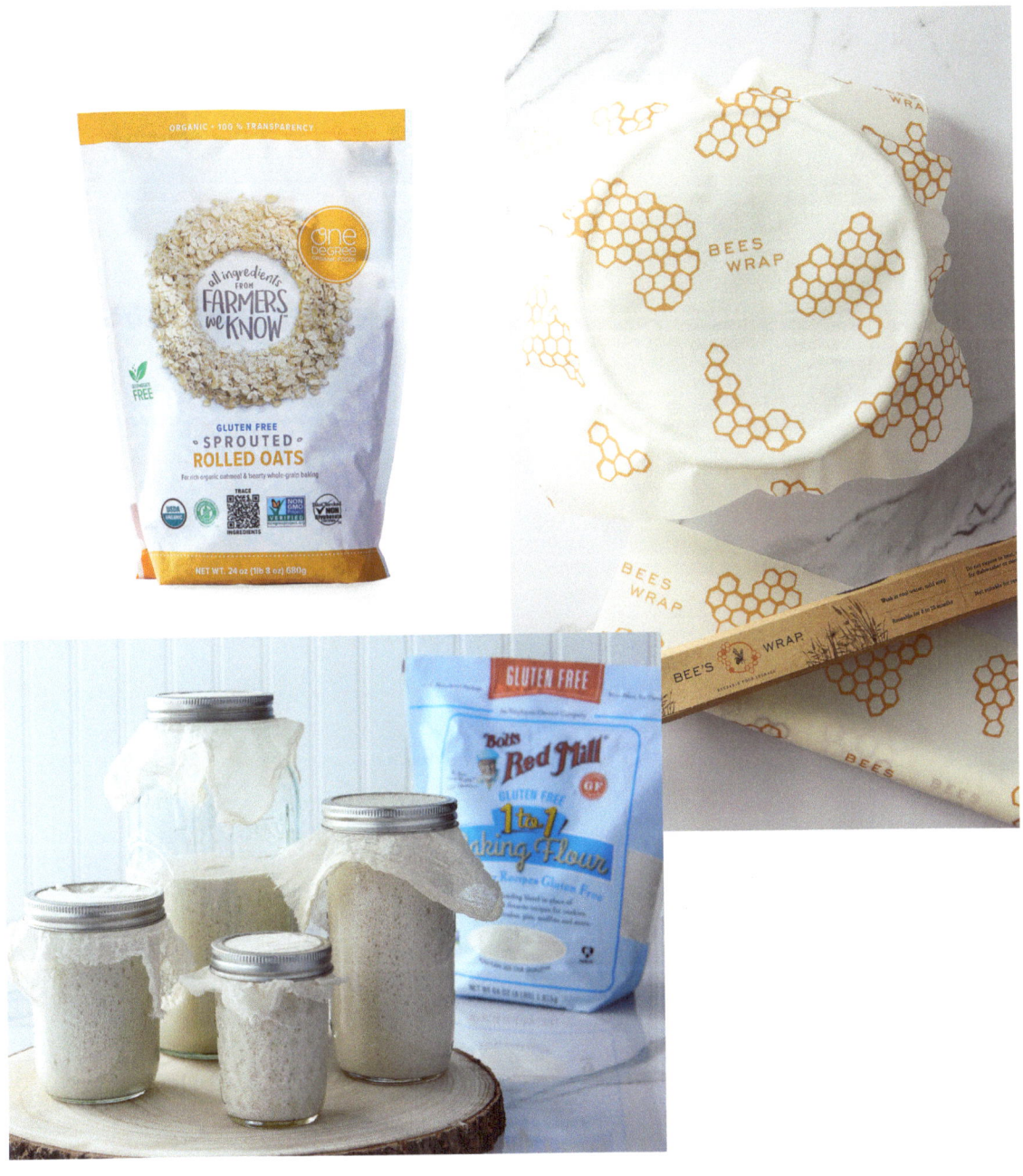

About the Author

Kasey Lobb is a self-professed food nerd, registered dietitian nutritionist, plant-based chef and passionate gluten-free baker. Most days, you'll find her in the kitchen experimenting with a new recipe and tending to her *mother*, her gluten-free sourdough starter. Over the past 20 years, Kasey has dedicated her career to helping people transform their health through food, specializing in food sensitivities and autoimmune diseases.

For two decades in her private practice, she worked with patients to manage inflammation and rediscover their vitality through specialized and elimination diets. Having personally navigated gluten and dairy sensitivities, Kasey knows the importance of healing the body while still enjoying food. Whether she's baking a loaf of gluten-free sourdough, teaching cooking classes or creating nourishing meals for her family, cooking gluten- and dairy-free is her passion.

Kasey holds a Bachelor of Science degree in Nutrition and Dietetics and a Master of Science degree in Dietetics and Institutional Administration, both from Texas Woman's University. She is a Registered and Licensed Dietitian Nutritionist with Advanced Certificate of Training in Adult Weight Management through the Academy of Nutrition and Dietetics. Kasey is also a Certified Lifestyle Eating and Performance Therapist, specializing in treating inflammatory food reactions.

Kasey is a certified plant-based chef and has trained at cooking schools around the world, including Costa Rica, France, Israel, Ireland, Italy, Turkey and the USA. Over the years, she has honed her cooking skills and deepened her passion for living a gluten- and dairy-free lifestyle. This journey inspired her to launch Appetite to Travel, LLC and begin writing cookbooks.

The Gluten-Free Sourdough Cookbook: gluten-free and dairy-free recipes for everyday baking marks a stirring new chapter in Kasey's personal and professional journey. Her goal is to empower anyone to bake with confidence, using accessible ingredients to create nourishing foods that the whole family will love.

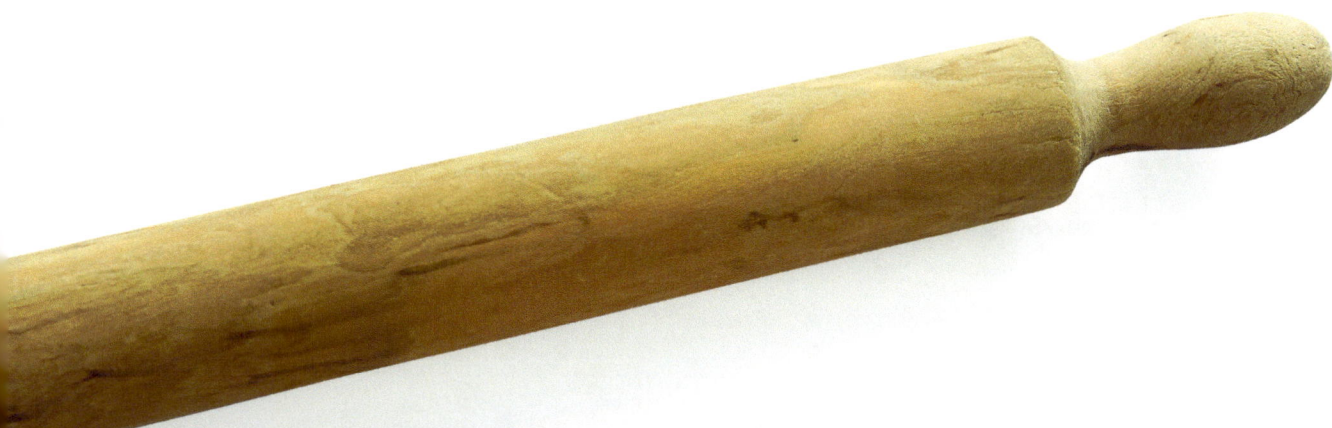

Index

Notes

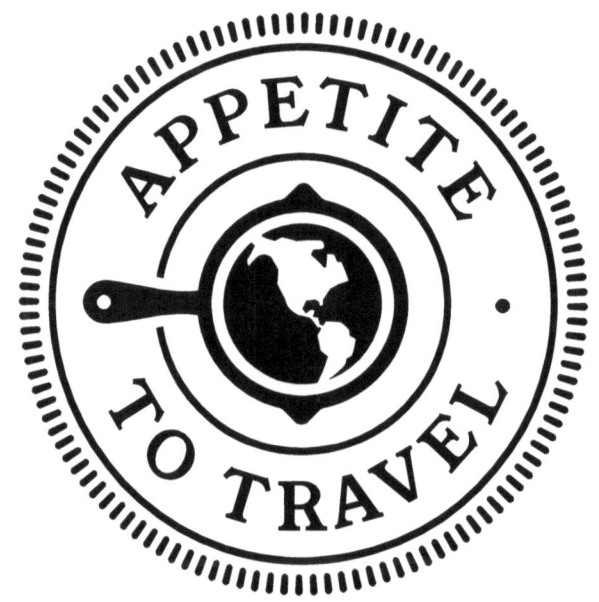

Appetite to Travel, LLC was created in 2019 by a culinary registered dietitian
nutritionist and a medical doctor, supported by a wonderful team of
travel agents, food advisors, interns and graphic designer.

We believe gathering around the table is a living symbol of culture, family and friendship,
and all are welcome. We look forward to breaking (gluten-free) bread with you!

For the latest on our books, classes and tours, please visit our website.

www.AppetiteToTravel.com

www.ingramcontent.com/pod-product-compliance
Lightning Source LLC
Chambersburg PA
CBHW041455120626
46547CB00003B/444